Odyssey of Hearing Loss

Tales of Triumph

Odyssey of Hearing Loss

Tales of Triumph

Michael A. Harvey

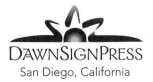

DawnSignPress

San Diego, California

Producer: Joe Dannis
Manufactured in the United States of America.
Published by DawnSignPress.

The information contained in this book is intended to be educational and not for
diagnosis, prescription, or treatment of health disorders, whatsoever. This information should not replace competent medical care. The Author and Publisher are in
no way liable for any use or misuse of the information.

Library of Congress Cataloging-in-Publication Data

Harvey, Michael A.
     Odyssey of hearing loss: tales of triumph / Michael A. Harvey.
       p. cm.
     Originally published: c1998.
     ISBN 0-58121-007-8 (pbk: alk. paper)
        1. Hearing impaired—United States—Psychology—Case studies. 2. Deaf—
     United States—Psychology—Cases studies. 3. Postlingual deafness—United
     States—Psychological aspects—Case studies. 4. Psychotherapy—United States
     —Case studies. I. Title.

     HV2545.H39 2003
     362.4'2'092273—dc21

                                                                            2003055251

ATTENTION:

Quantity discounts for schools, bookstores, and
distributors are available.

For information, please contact:

DAWNSIGNPRESS
6130 Nancy Ridge Drive
San Diego, CA 92121
619-625-0600 V/VP 619-625-2336 FAX
ORDER TOLL FREE 1-800-549-5350
www.dawnsign.com

For Janet, Allison, and Emily

Contents

Acknowledgments

First, I would like to express my deep gratitude to the people whose stories are in this book. The names and details of each tale have been changed to protect confidentiality. Each person reviewed the manuscript, found the material to be sufficiently disguised, and gave written consent for the material's publication.

Marylyn Howe has been a constant source of inspirational support. Her detailed and erudite feedback has been invaluable.

My sincere thanks and appreciation goes to my colleagues Ben Bahan and Robert Hoffmeister, and to my mother, Barbara Hamburg, for their support and editorial suggestions. My father, Harmond Harvey, read the entire book and gave me copious notes and cogent ideas.

It was my good fortune to work with DawnSignPress. Beginning with the support and enthusiasm of Joe Dannis, I have thoroughly appreciated working with Rebecca Ryan and her production staff.

Finally, it seems somehow significant to me that DawnSignPress received the completed book manuscript on the day of Marie Jean Philip's funeral. As she was with so many others throughout the world, Marie was a cherished mentor to me. She never grew tired of challenging me in supportive and respectful ways, albeit with sometimes painful honesty. Perhaps like many others, I never told her just how grateful and honored I was for her wisdom and help.

Introduction

When I first learned about psychological adjustment to acquired hearing loss, it all seemed so clear and self-evident. The stages of adjustment could be listed, the positive and negative ways of coping could be catalogued, and clear recommendations could be made. I imagined a late-deafened person coming to psychotherapy and a therapist diagnosing the problem, making well-targeted interventions, and finding a solution. A neat package.

On one hand, I often long for that early clarity, but on the other hand, I am grateful for the growth offered by the not-so-clear reality. Human beings are simple only at a distance. Bearing witness to our multidimensional complexity frees us from the objectification of stereotypes, theories, and textbooks. If, by some magical power, we were able to render another's personal story as self-evident, predictable, and measurable, then life would lose luminosity and its power to teach about purpose, loss, transition, and spirituality. This book continues a long tradition of attempting to understand human existence, not with neat-packaged answers (there are often no answers at all), but with stories.

Most of the stories are about people who defined themselves from an audiological perspective as having experienced a reduction or loss of hearing. Rather than identify with the Deaf community and Deaf culture, they labeled themselves as having an "acquired hearing loss" or as "hard-of-hearing," "deafened," "hearing-impaired," or "deaf."* None of them were born deaf. Most used English as their primary language—not a signed language—and most reported feeling more comfortable at Association of Late-Deafened Adults (A.L.D.A.) or Self Help for the Hard of Hearing (S.H.H.H.) gatherings than at Deaf community gatherings.

All of the people in these stories were confronted, to different degrees, by stigma, by assaults to their self-esteem and self-determination, by threatened isolation, by helpful and nonhelpful reactions of family and friends, by often conflicting professional guidance, and by spiritual crises.

Beyond these commonalties, there were also many differences. Most had requested psychotherapy themselves, but others like Norma and Steven were "dragged" to my office. Carol was a pen pal and not a client at all. Their hearing loss was also varied. Robert experienced a sudden, severe hearing loss as a young child; Mary first noticed her progressive hearing loss as an adolescent; Donna, as a young adult. Norma suffered from presbycusis, which started in her late sixties. Ann, unlike any of the others in this book, considered herself culturally Deaf and was a fluent user of American Sign Language. Jason complained not of his mild hearing loss, but of tinnitus (ringing in the ears). While Steven would do anything to get rid of his progressive hearing loss and was even investigating cochlear implants, Eric was grateful for having become deaf, as it furthered his spiritual growth.

My Own Story

The therapist is not only witness to another's story, but also inevitably a participant. As a more personal way of intro-

---

*The uncapitalized deaf refers to those who, from an audiological perspective, view themselves as having a profound hearing loss but who choose not to be culturally Deaf. Deaf (with a capital D) refers to culturally Deaf people.

ducing how and why I began to work with people with hearing loss, I include my own story.

First of all, I am hearing. I have no deaf or hard-of-hearing family members. Growing up, I had never met anyone with a significant hearing loss. My entry into the field of working with deaf people dates back to 1979 when the Mayor and Selectman of San Francisco were murdered. I attended a lecture by a psychiatrist who vehemently attacked the diminished capacity claim of the defense. However, I found myself captivated, not so much by the subject matter, but by the sign language interpreter who was there for the deaf members of the audience.

Later that week, I came across an advertisement for an American Sign Language (ASL) course at a nearby college. It looked intriguing. ASL would be a different kind of hobby, one that would balance my life, which at that time was too filled with academic and professional demands. I soon found myself sitting second row center in an ASL class taught by a Deaf teacher.

Like many others who first encounter the Deaf world, I felt like I was beamed down to another planet, one with its own language, culture, and set of customs. My intrigue and fascination propelled me to practice sign language with the hope of being able to hold a respectable conversation with the Deaf people I would meet.

On a deeper level, obviously there were other reasons for my continued intrigue. One was an appreciation of the richness of many deaf peoples' lives despite society's denigration of them. I felt privileged to observe close-at-hand their strength in the face of oppression, which manifested as job discrimination, subtle and overt bigotry, negative stereotyping, and humiliation. Many transformed what could have been the irrevocably toxic effects of that oppression into a sense of purpose and depth. I am continually amazed how crises have a way of crushing or strengthening the human spirit. In the words of African-American author and poet Maya Angelou

> You may shoot me with your words,
> You may cut me with your eyes,
> You may kill me with your hatefulness,
> But still, like air, I'll rise.[1]

Looking back, I realize that in addition to the novelty and appreciation of their strength, meeting deaf and hard-of-hearing people inspired me. There is hope! I, too, can overcome whatever adversities come my way. Perhaps at some level of consciousness I thought they would share their secret with me about the necessary ingredients for resilience. I would somehow absorb their wisdom.

In terms of my own experiences, I have never personally incurred any significant degree of oppression. However, as a Jew, I have always been affected by the Holocaust and other acts of anti-Semitism. Six years after my Bar Mitzvah, I wrote in my diary:

> I'm not Jewish. Why would I want to join a team that has a record of 6 million losses?

I had remained steadfast in renouncing my Jewish identity until thirty years later when my then seven-year-old daughter asked to enter Hebrew school, admittedly to be with her friends. What do I tell her? After much introspection, I told Allison that we would join a temple and learn about Judaism together. I privately decided it was time to come to terms with the Holocaust and with God. The God whom I thought had let the genocide happen.

My next step was to come to terms with those who were closest to the "final solution." I joined a German-Jewish dialogue group. The German participants were mostly related to Nazi perpetrators and the Jewish participants were mostly survivors of the Holocaust.

During one meeting, a key question came up: What do we need from each other? As a Jew, what do I "need" from the Germans to heal my psychic wounds? What might they "need" from me? I learned an important lesson: I needed empathy and validation from both groups. The support I needed from other Jews felt self-evident and comfortable. With the Germans, however, I felt a strange sense of terror and rage, coupled with an almost inexplicable need for their emotional validation. It was this duality of feelings that I needed the Germans to understand.

I also needed to visit the Auschwitz Memorial in Poland. I will never forget standing at the center of Auschwitz—in the midst of the nihilistic void. Even while wondering what would become of our species given the enormity of the horror and tragedy that had happened there, I noticed what still felt alive in the environment: the beautiful landscape, the trees, and the lakes. Many German people were praying and crying. I felt that I understood some of their pain and that they understood some of mine. Then that place became sacred for me. I stood silent for a long while.

I have always been intrigued by the inherent benefits of respectful dialogue between oppressed and oppressor groups: Jewish and German; Deaf and Hearing. In the German-Jewish group I came to have compassion for how the German participants also felt terror, rage, and/or shame about the Nazi regime. After more extended dialogue (several years of monthly meetings), I could no longer fit us into discrete categories of either victims or victimizers. At different levels, we were both. Through dialogue with Deaf persons, I have also gotten a glimpse of the duality of good and evil in all persons, including myself. Rather than taking the comfortable but naive position that "I never oppress," I now ask "under what conditions am I likely to oppress and to what degree?" Here, too, discrete categories of me and them disappear.

Alexander Solzhenitsyn said it best:

If only it were all so simple! If only there were evil
people somewhere insidiously committing evil
deeds, and it were necessary only to separate them
from the rest of us and destroy them. But the line
dividing good and evil cuts through the heart of
every human being. And who is willing to destroy a
piece of his own heart?[2]

These are parts of my own life story that resonate when
I work with deaf persons. Because of these experiences—
and undoubtedly others that are beyond my awareness—
the "just one sign language course" became several and
much more than a hobby. Later I became director of
D.E.A.F, Inc., a nonprofit community-based agency in All-
ston, Massachusetts, began a private psychotherapy and
consultation practice, then became an adjunct professor at
Boston University Center for the Study of Communication
and the Deaf, taught two courses at Gallaudet University's
Department of Counseling and, most recently, became adjunct faculty at Pennsylvania College of Optometry, School
of Audiology.

Strange as it may seem, my life is based on a true story.[3]

In its essence, this book is a collection of the tales of
people who have acquired hearing losses. As such, they may
be true or false when compared to the tales of many others.
Statistically speaking, the people in this book may not be a
representative sample of the general population. That is,
some may nod their heads in agreement, saying "Yeah,
that's how I feel, too!" and others may shake their heads,
saying "[Jason/Sue/Carol/Robert] may have felt so and so,
but not me!"

This level of analysis misses the point for no two people
have the same story. Yet any two stories may be common

enough to inspire a dialogue and discover an oasis of essential alikeness amidst the hearing world which doesn't understand. If all of the people in this book could somehow meet, my bet is that they would share their unique sensitivities to issues of conversational accessibility and the need for assertiveness, educating others, and maintaining their pride and self esteem. My fantasy is that they would forbid outsiders—hearing people—to attend the group meeting. As Carol in the final chapter states, "you have to be deafened to understand."

At the same time, however, different stories resonate with each other, providing a glimpse of humanity. Many of us have had the experience of beginning relationships, thinking we are bound by our own separate stories. With a sense of humility and awe, we learn again and again that strange as it may seem the milestones and transformations of our lives are indeed based on universally true stories that have been recorded throughout the history of humankind.

In summary, *Odyssey of Hearing Loss: Tales of Triumph* is a testament of how various individuals attempted to answer the questions that their hearing loss had forced on them. It is also a testament of my successful and futile struggles to answer the questions asked of me by those who sought my help. Sometimes, I felt confident, on safe ground, and proud of my clinical acumen; other times, I felt disoriented and adrift.

For me, while the triumphs contained in our life odysseys are no longer surprising, they continue to be profoundly amazing and inspiring. For that I am grateful.

———

I would appreciate feedback and questions from readers. Please write to me, c/o DawnSignPress, 6130 Nancy Ridge Drive, San Diego, California, 92121-3223. Or send e-mail to comments@dawnsign.com. Make sure you include the book's title on the subject line.

Notes

1. Angelou, M. (1978). *Still I rise.* New York: Random House.

2. Zweig, C. and Abrams, J. (1991). *Meeting the shadow.* New York: Putnam.

3. This quote cited from a web site (1998). Ashleigh Brillant. http//www.chesco.com/~artman/brilliant.hmtl.

A Framework

One day I couldn't start my car. "Just once," my mechanic begged, "why can't someone bring me a car that's running well?"

"What would be the point?" I replied.

He grunted. "I guess it's like people who are happy and fulfilled coming to see you, huh?"

Whereas my mechanic is an expert at fixing cars, he exemplifies a common misconception with regard to psychotherapy. I happily do not view myself as psychologically "repairing" those who come to my office to get them "running well." The "broken" metaphor works well with engines, but is simplistic and dehumanizing when applied to people. There is a subtle but important distinction between certifying a person as maladjusted, or broken, and helping someone gain self-understanding and enrichment.

One of my roles as a psychotherapist is to discover and illuminate certain universal truths on which clients' lives are based, to assist that truth-telling process, and to bear witness to the profound joys and anguishes that are revealed. Our collaboration can be described as an archeological dig of sorts, whereby we excavate and examine what lays beneath the seemingly uniform, even surfaces of their tales: fear, despair, fortitude, contentment, and spirituality, to mention only a few artifacts. Through our dialogue, we discover their

1

dark caves and dragons as well as pockets of gold—universal dualities of lightness and darkness, and complex truths. Finally, I step back and attempt to make sense of it all.

But then things become more complex. The stories in this book force us to acknowledge one fundamental difference between humans and car engines. Unlike engines, we do not come with specification manuals. There is no objective method of completely understanding human beings. Instead, we can rely only on peoples' tales, their personal narratives.

This book offers a psycho–social–spiritual framework in which to understand the personal narratives of hard-of-hearing people and those with acquired hearing loss. It chronicles how psychological, social, and spiritual factors are interwoven, shaping the life stories of ten people, and how understanding these factors through psychotherapy gives clients insight into how to improve their lives.

A Psycho–Social–Spiritual Framework

Psycho. Human beings have an inner psychology. We experience an endless stream of conscious and unconscious thoughts, feelings, and impulses. We can define "parts" of our psyche as conscious and unconscious, rational and irrational, id–ego–superego, the "inner child," etc.

Social. In addition, we are social creatures, products of overlapping social networks. The reactions of other people, significant others, parents, families, friends, neighbors, teachers, bosses, professional helpers, remain important influences on our lives. In the words of seventeenth century English poet John Donne, "No man is an island entire of itself; every man is part of the main."

Spiritual. Unlike the "psycho-social" parts which can be clearly defined, the definition of spiritual is anything but clear. In the chapter titled "Resilience to Trauma: An Inspirational Voice from Cyberspace," Carol defines her spirituality as "feeling like everything's connected; like I'm part of a larger whole." Others believe in "a power beyond us, an organizing principle." In the popular movie, "Star Wars," Obi-Wan Kenobi blessed Luke Skywalker with "May the force be with you." And 12-step programs teach about "the higher power."

Perhaps as human beings we are wired to at least consider the question of whether there is some undefinable power or energy beyond us.[1] In fact, it is often in elementary school that we first begin to wonder whether there is a God; and if so, what is "it."[2] As adults, we often continue to ask ourselves that question, particularly in times surrounding a crisis or major loss.

There are many possible answers to the God question. What answer we choose strongly influences the way we interpret our experience. During a coffee break from writing this chapter, I happened to come across an article in the local Boston newspaper entitled "Spirituality Makes Rounds." It described "new areas of inquiry" for physicians doing medical rounds at Massachusetts General Hospital.

> We need to go to patients and see what they see as spirituality. Very often that takes away the conflict between spirituality and medicine; they don't have to be in opposition.[3]

Therefore, although spirituality is difficult to define, and each person must ultimately define spirituality for themselves, it is a pervasive part of human existence.

Psychological, social, and spiritual factors influence the way one perceives any event,* and a psycho–social–spiritual framework is useful in understanding how people experience acquired hearing loss.

---

*Although biological factors are obviously also important, their inclusion is beyond the scope of this book.

Trauma and Triumph

I was initially hesitant to describe adventitious hearing loss as potentially traumatic. Trauma evokes images of war, rape, abuse, helplessness, victimization, and frailty. It is a psychiatric label and implicitly connotes psychiatric maladjustment, suggesting that there is something mentally wrong or deficient about the traumatized individual. Trauma then creates a potential industry of "helpers," who earn their living "helping," whether or not the individual wants or needs their help.

Many deafened people rightly claim that they have enough to worry about without professionals imposing a diagnosis on them. They ask "Why not refer to the *impact* of hearing loss, the *stress* of hearing loss, or its positive and negative effects?" "Anything but trauma."

There are others, however, who feel invalidated at the suggestion that hearing loss is anything less than potentially traumatic. They understand the label of trauma not as demeaning and pathological, but as a validation of their experiences. For them, trauma is more a restoration of their dignity following verbal assaults from others such as "don't be lazy," "you should try harder," or "stop feeling sorry for yourself," and they feel justified about needing time and support to heal.

Unlike many congenitally deaf and hard-of-hearing persons whose level of hearing has become an integral facet of their identity, people who once had hearing experience a loss of a sensory capacity with which they had defined themselves. Holly Elliot, a social worker who became deaf, emphasized that "prelingual deafness is a sensory deficit. Acquired deafness is a sensory deprivation."[4] Similarly, British Parliament member Jack Ashley—himself deafened—observed that "the born deaf are denied the advantages gained by the deafened before their hearing loss, yet they are spared the desolating sense of loss."[5]

Ashley listed adjectives about his own sudden hearing loss: "thunderbolt of deafness," "tortured months," "shattering beyond belief," "plummeting of my happiness, aspirations, and hopes for the future," and "existing in misery."[6] Another deafened man echoed that "my hearing loss is like an emptiness, a vacuum, a pit."

A forty-year-old woman described a recurring dream which began soon after she woke up one morning profoundly deaf.

> It was a cool, sunny day in California. I was running in a field with a group of friends, laughing and singing. All of a sudden, there was a huge earthquake. The sky turned black, the ground opened up, and I fell in head first, tumbling down.

To summarize the above reactions—and many of the tales in this book—as simply indicative of stress or, on the other hand, as "blessings in disguise" is inadequate at best, disrespectful at worst.

We have very personal relationships with language, particularly when it comes to describing our own experiences. For example, a hard-of-hearing man sent me the following response in reaction to an article I had written on the psychological pain of hearing loss: "This letter is to let you know how I feel about using the word 'pain' for this and that and everything. . . . There is no pain with hearing loss. Misery, yes."

One person's pain is another's misery; one's trauma is another's stress is another's challenge. Call it what you will. Why is the label so important?

The implications of deeming acquired hearing loss as potentially traumatic go beyond satisfying personal language preference. It helps us acknowledge the many subtle and overt ripple effects that hearing loss may have on one's psyche. In psychiatrist Judith Herman's words, "The label of trauma honors one's experience instead of de-meaning it."[7]

The Process of Psychotherapy

Although many of the people in this book initially requested psychotherapy only to "feel better"—for me to somehow extract their distress by performing a "distress-ectomy"—our dialogue would inevitably illuminate how that goal did not represent triumph. Triumph over loss does not mean winning, living happily ever after (as in old Walt Disney movies), "getting over it," or the guarantee of no more suffering. Even in cases of so-called "complete" recovery from a serious physical illness or the loss of health, there are permanent psychological remnants or scar tissue which can cast both ominous shadows and illuminate growth opportunities.

It is not the case that clients simply reveal themselves during the therapy hour. By necessity, the lens I use to understand and shape another's story is shaped by my own story—influenced not only by my formal clinical training, but also by my own personal development. As in the case of Norma and her family in the chapter titled "Presbycusis, Mortality, and Brussels Sprouts," it was only when I could allow myself to at least begin facing my own mortality that I could tolerate Norma telling her children how she wanted to live and to die. Before I got my act together, my own issues suffocated her story.

A client's story inevitably influences my own; it is not a one-way street. I, too, benefit from the therapeutic dialogue. In the chapter titled "Tinnitus No More: Aspen Here I Come" the eternal moment when Jason clasped my hands to reduce the loneliness of his suffering is forever etched in my mind. That moment is one of many similar moments in my work that have given texture to my life.

Most of these clients were also pleased with the significant improvements in their lives which, by design, were attributable to therapy. However, such improvements were never guaranteed. Instead, independent of any symptom-relief outcome, each client inevitably became increasingly more responsible for his or her existence. That is the guaranteed outcome of successful therapy.

Through therapy, identifying a person's particular combination of *validating* and *invalidating* psychological, social, and spiritual factors can guide them to view their hearing loss as a "deficit to be corrected or a difference to be accepted."[8]

Hearing loss as a deficit to be corrected. When people define themselves as inadequate and deficient purportedly because of their hearing loss, it is not because of their hearing loss per se. One's self-definition is never made in isolation. A person's psychological feelings of inferiority are, in fact, a social construction; these feelings mirror society's negative view that having a hearing deficit prevents one from living a full life.[9] The false idea is that deaf people need help from hearing professionals to be successful and cope with stresses in the hearing world.[10]

The ramifications of the so-called medical or pathological perspective of deafness are both severely debilitating and oppressive. Several professional texts, for example, describe in pejorative terms "the psychology of deafness"—essentially that a deaf person's psyche "doesn't work right" or that it is "broken." This notion is really more about the psychology of many hearing professionals who try to help deaf people think, feel, and behave like hearing people.[11,12]

This pathological stance can pollute one's spirituality. In the chapter titled "Pockets of Gold," Eric's initial response to his hearing loss was "Why should I say 'Amen' at church? An almighty God wouldn't inflict deafness on me like this!" From that moment on, Eric had dismissed God as nonexistent, as dead. Variations of this spiritual crisis are common, particularly for those who believe in a benevolent, omnipotent, and omniscient God.[13]

Hearing loss as a difference to be accepted. There are other more affirming possibilities for how to define one's acquired hearing loss. As an example, Carol (Resilience to Trauma: An Inspirational Voice from Cyberspace) forged a balance between loss and growth proving that "acquired hearing loss does not mean succumbing to an unfulfilled life." With the support of her family, and building on her inner strength, Carol met life's challenges head on, maintaining a professional life in the hearing world and also becoming involved in organizations for late-deafened adults and in Deaf culture.

The Association of Late-Deafened Adults (A.L.D.A.) and Self Help for the Hard of Hearing (S.H.H.H.) are examples of affirmative social networks. Many persons with acquired hearing loss describe their annual meetings as a kind of going home. As one woman put it,

> At A.L.D.A., I'm no longer alone nor handicapped. I'm accepted for who I am by my peers. It may sound funny, but going to the meetings has also been a kind of spiritual journey for me. I feel a connection to something larger than all of us.

The Deaf Cultural Movement is another example of an affirmative stance of empowerment against the predominant pathological perspective.[14] The cohesiveness of the Deaf community heals the wounds which are the result of many hearing professionals' attempts to eradicate deafness. As such, Deaf culture is an extremely positive phenomenon that affirms and validates a Deaf person's sense of self.

Therapist Lessons

To the best of my ability, I avoid participating in society's insidious denigration of deaf people. My therapeutic agenda is to help an individual sort out the multilayered psychological, social, and spiritual influences that have often unknowingly shaped his or her existence, and then to help that person live a more fulfilled life. *Easier said than done.*

It is the client who begins the dialogue with his or her own story. Then the therapist. Soon, however, these two stories resonate to become a new, combined story—one that is more evolved than what could have been produced solely by either party. This is the magic of intimate dialogue. It is the means par excellence of learning life's important and sacred lessons.

One lesson I have learned is that every human experience can be expressed in terms of a paradox. As an example, a person's unique complexity can coexist with that person also echoing a universal theme: "I am both the same as and different from other people." The tales in this book document an omnipresent tension encompassed in that particular/universal duality, namely, that persons with acquired hearing loss have experiences that are both unique to themselves and humanly comprehensive.

With the acknowledgment of duality, things do not seem so either/or, positive/negative anymore. Rather, the Yin and Yang combine to form a whole. F. Scott Fitzgerald referred to the experience of accepting duality as "holding two opposed ideas at the same time, and still retaining the ability to function." Psychiatrist Carl Jung referred to this process as "the union of opposites."

Do persons with acquired hearing loss tolerate their hurt, then grieve, cope and do the best they can? Or do they reap the benefits and rejoice? It may be that they do both. To be whole, we have to integrate the myriad dualities which characterize human existence.

Synchronicity is another frequent theme in this book. It is always awe-inspiring to experience those meaningful coincidences—when events happen together seemingly accidentally, but really as if "something else" is going on. In the chapter "Presbycusis, Mortality, and Brussels Sprouts" Marty happens to fall down his basement stairs just at the right time to help his mother examine her own mortality in family therapy. In the chapter "Dear Mom and Dad, if Only You Had Known," Sue happens to find her late mother's diary as a final step toward reconciling their relationship. There are many such examples.

Somehow everything is connected. I'm just not sure how. What once seemed so simple ain't. Instead, in the words of the wise Mystics, we are surrounded by a "cloud of unknowingness."

———

I wanted to tell all of this to my mechanic. But I was already late for an appointment. I gave him this chapter instead.

Notes

1. Armstong, K. (1993). *A history of God*. New York: Ballantine Books.

2. Coles, R. (1991). *The spiritual life of children*. New York: Houghton Mifflin.

3. Tye, L. (1997, November 4). *Spirituality makes rounds*. Boston Globe.

4. Elliot, H. (1986). *Acquired deafness: Shifting gears*. Speech delivered at a workshop for deafened adults. San Francisco, CA.

5. Ashley, J. (1985). "Deafness in the family." In H. Orlans (Ed.). *Adjustment to adult hearing loss*. San Diego, CA: College-Hill Press.

6. Ashley, "Deafness in the family."

7. Herman, J. L. (1992). *Trauma and recovery*. New York: Basic Books.

8. Freeman, R. D., Carbin, C. F., & Boese, R. J. (1981). *Can't your child hear? A guide for those who care about deaf children*. Baltimore, MD: University Park Press.

9. Lane, H. (1984). *When the mind hears: A history of the deaf.* New York: Random House.

10. Lane, H., Hoffmeister, R., & Bahan, B. (1996). *A journey into the deaf–world.* San Diego: DawnSignPress.

11. Lane, H. (1992). *The mask of benevolence.* San Diego: DawnSignPress.

12. Hoffmeister, R. J., & Harvey, M. A. (1997). Is there a psychology of the hearing? In N. Glickman & M. A. Harvey (Eds.), *Culturally affirmative psychotherapy with deaf people.* New Jersey: Lawrence Erlbaum Associates.

13. Kushner, H. (1981). *When bad things happen to good people.* New York: Avon Publishers.

14. Lane, Hoffmeister, & Bahan. *Journey into the deaf–world.*

Dear Mom and Dad, if Only You Had Known

Before I could even say hello, Sue told me that she didn't want to be here.

"It may sound silly," she began, "but I just got a letter from my mom. She went on and on about volunteering at the hospital, planting carrots in her garden, and other stuff like our neighbor's son getting an award and Dad buying a new lawn mower."

I could not help but be tempted to ask her what kind of mower he had bought (as mine had just broke), but now was not the appropriate time for humor. She looked more disheveled than usual and her eyes were puffy, as if she had been crying. Given her statement that she did not want to come, it was odd that she arrived unusually early for her appointment. It didn't add up. I also could not figure out why her Mom's letter was so upsetting.

Sue had requested psychotherapy about four months prior because she wanted to "like herself more as a hard-of-hearing person." She often felt inadequate when attempting to learn new computer programming languages at work, was trying to figure out how to take care of her own emotional needs without "supporting the whole world," and sometimes felt unfulfilled in her marriage. Now in her early forties, she wondered what more there was to life.

We had spent a lot of time separating common hearing loss issues, such as the daily communication challenges, from universal "problems in living." For the most part, Sue and I ended up agreeing that she suffered from those inevitable life struggles that beset all of us. We also agreed that she was overattributing her difficulties to her hearing loss. Depending on the day, she viewed everyday life difficulties as either opportunities or irritants. We have all been there.

On our seventh visit, Sue announced that she had put her complaints in perspective and wished to terminate therapy. She and her husband had just gone to Cape Cod for a "wonderful, connecting weekend" and she had restructured her schedule to make time for herself. She enrolled in a meditation class and a Greek cooking class—"That'll take care of my mind and stomach," she joked. We planned to say goodbye.

Today, however, the quality of her sadness and anger was different. Her feelings did not seem so much a byproduct of present-day frustrations, but rather seemed interwoven in early childhood memories. The card from her mother had catapulted Sue backward in time to when her hearing loss—diagnosed at the age of five due to meningitis—helped create a rift between Sue and her parents.

"Her card made me think about how I never quite felt included at home," Sue began. "My Mom and Dad would often mumble and expect me to figure out what was going on. But worst of all, it was taboo to talk about how I felt! Nobody wanted to listen. They knew I could lip-read well so it was no big deal! And when I wanted to talk about my hearing loss, my Mom would dismiss me with 'You do know, dear, you have a hearing loss which means you need to try harder but you are just like everyone else so don't worry about it and now please finish your peas and then help me clean up and then we'll go. . . .' Like in her card, Mom would ramble on and say absolutely nothing!"

Her comments about her mother revealed her anger, but anger soon gave way to renewed tears. Finally, she stared into empty space and in a soft, frail voice she said, "If my mother were only here now!"

I instinctively asked her if she would like to invite her mother to come in for a meeting. Without hesitation, however, she shook her head no and said that both her parents had serious health problems and that she didn't want to upset them.

If they could not literally join our meeting, maybe we could in fantasy bring the past into the present. So I asked Sue to talk to her mom as if she were in the office. I motioned to an empty seat.

Sue's countenance immediately changed, her eyes became dilated and she sat up in her seat. "You mean talk to my Mom now?" she asked in confusion.

"Better late than never," I affirmed. "Besides, it's just make-believe. She's not really here."

She needed no more coaxing. I watched as Sue visually placed her mom on the empty chair. Then she nervously grimaced and looked back at me for support. I nodded my head. After a moment of staring at her imagined mother, her nostrils flared up and she gritted her teeth. After a few slow, deep breaths, Sue began a long overdue proclamation: "Mom, stop it!" she started off meekly and paused. "Stop! STOP!! [now louder] I'll eat the damn peas! I'll help you clean. [pause] Do you know I'm sinking fast? What should I do? I'm scared. When I go to school, I'm alone— in a capsule away from the teacher, away from everyone else. Like you keep telling me to do, I try real hard to be part of things, but I can't! Everything feels fuzzy and I disappear. And I don't know why. Do you understand? Do you understand?"

Whereas she began with indignant anger, she ended with despair. As we discussed what lay beneath her anger and despair, Sue got in touch with her long-buried need for emotional acknowledgment and validation, particularly from her mother. It was a thwarted need that both parties had long since dismissed as "no big deal" and even as "baby-ish." But it left an emptiness in Sue—in her words, "an inner hollowness." As a child, Sue would eat those "damn peas" and help with what inevitably were endless family chores which would distract her from these feelings. And as an adult, she would overeat and work longer hours.

Her need for validation was, in fact, not babyish at all. For all of us that need begins in infancy and continues through mature adulthood. Just as kids often stare at themselves in mirrors, their physical sense of self is defined by the mirrored reflections. How else can they know what they look like? Similarly, our psychological sense of self is de-fined vis-á-vis "psychological mirrors" in the form of other people. We grow in connection with significant others. We all have what are called mirroring needs.[1]

Without acknowledgment and validation from another, we cannot develop a strong psychological sense of self. As Sue reminisced, "I never knew how I felt because I couldn't tell anyone."

Sue, like many people, did not rest easy with the idea that her private sense of self was dependent upon her relation-ships with other people. Yet even astronauts, chosen for their fortitude, sense of purpose, and intelligence, must accept this fact. In the isolation of space, they must depend on rou-tines, tasks, and orders from earthbound command centers to keep their orientation and to resist the pull of merger and fragmentation resulting in loss of self. Underwater divers must take similar precautions.[2] Without an external relation-ship with another person to compare and differentiate one-self, there is no self-definition, no stable sense of reality.

As Sue and I continued to examine the quality of her previous relationships, she commented, "As far back as I can remember," she began, "there has always been fuzziness between me and other people. It was as if I walked around asleep all the time."

I was struck by her choice of the words "fuzziness" and "asleep." I wondered aloud whether the analogies of astronauts or underwater divers fit. Whether her alienation from her parents and peers—due to their failure to adequately mirror her experience of hearing loss—set the stage for her feeling alienated internally. Psychiatrist Heinz Kohut aptly termed this experience "fragmentation of self."[3] It is like a shattered mirror.

After a moment, Sue nodded in agreement: "When my brother and sister bragged about what they had learned in school, I wanted to brag, too. But I had nothing to brag about. I thought I was stupid or lazy. My dad always asked me how school was and I automatically replied 'fine.' I couldn't tell him that going to school was like drowning in ice water. I got so good at bluffing my way through everything that I forgot who I was. Or maybe I never knew? And nobody noticed. I felt like a person who was not a 'real' person. Like I didn't exist 'as much' as everyone else. That's the story of my life! Now, I have trouble figuring out what I need. How I feel. Who I am. I never really know if I am really enjoying a relationship or if I'm just making sure that the other person enjoys me and thinks I'm normal. I am who you want me to be! My fear of being left out, nonexistent, and invisible makes me feel an urgent, overpowering need to participate in group meetings. I can then be counted as part of the human race! Then I will exist! But then comes the panic that I will be discovered as a charlatan, as someone bad or wrong. I'll be proven not to be a real person and will be kicked out of the world. I will die. In fact, I've always felt on the verge of dying."

I felt tempted at this point to comfort Sue, perhaps by commenting that she seemed very much alive as opposed to being on the verge of dying. But she had endured enough deflection of painful dialogue within her family and I did not want her to misunderstand my support as invalidating her feelings. She was bravely giving a voice to painful, previously "wordless" memories that had remained toxic in her life, precisely because they had been devoid of words. It was Nietzsche who said that "silence is poison."

I recalled a profound passage about grief: "You must not walk around the perimeter of loss. Instead, you must go through the center, grief's very core, in order to continue your own life in a meaningful way."[4] Sue was walking very much "toward the center" and my task was not to lead her astray. So I simply asked her to continue. After a moment or two of pensive silence, Sue replied: "I remember as a kid once standing in the dark barn looking out at the rectangle of light representing the outside world."

Her eyes gazed upward and I knew that she was back in the barn. Tears began streaming down her face and she hid her head in her lap. Her image was poignant, as it so aptly symbolized how one's definition of self is dependent on another. Where were her mother and father in her rectangle of light? How she had needed them to be there! Sue and her parents had spared themselves the "walk through grief's very core," but at what expense? Their silence had made their grief poisonous.

Thus began the next phase of our work. We would say goodbye later than we had planned. The next steps were clear. But our time had ended fifteen minutes ago. We had both lost track of the hour.

Sue arrived early again for our next appointment. This time she looked more anxious than sad. It felt different in the room, probably, I thought, because we had left familiar and safe territory and did not quite know what would come next.

My hunch was confirmed when she started the session with "I don't know what lies ahead."

"Christopher Columbus probably felt the same way," I offered.

This time some humor was called for and brought welcome respite from the anxiety of exploring the unfamiliar. Sue laughed and suggested we both take Dramamine to avoid seasickness.

I asked Sue for her thoughts and feelings about our last meeting. Before we continued walking through "grief's center," I wanted to make sure we were not going at too fast a pace.

"Well, to tell you the truth, I knew that my Mom's letter had struck a nerve and that I really needed to talk about it. Part of me was really looking forward to doing just that. But I was afraid you'd laugh at me, you know, for getting so upset about such a stupid letter."

"Like I would say 'don't worry about it, eat your peas' or something like that?"

"Yeah, I'm real sensitive to that."

"I can understand why. I know that your Mom's letter rubbed salt in some old wounds."

"Boy, that's an understatement. I woke up with hives the next morning. My doctor said it could have been stress related. And I haven't really slept well the last several nights."

After a short pause, I invited Sue to continue. She hesitated, I imagined, for fear I would dismiss her. She then made eye contact with me and said, "Well, you'll think this is crazy for sure, but I've been having really weird nightmares."

"Uh huh. Please go on." Another overture to continue.

"Last night I dreamt that I was walking through a forest when I tripped over some brush and fell into a mass grave! It was dark, cold, and completely silent. I was yelling for help but nobody was there. I woke up in a cold sweat, screaming."

Her earlier vision of "standing in the dark barn" seemed similar to her dream of falling in a dark grave. It made perfect sense, though, since "loss of self" is indeed a kind of psychological death. Her nightmare revealed her fears in their most unabashedly stark and uncensored form. Her daytime fantasy of the dark barn revealed the same fears but in a less frightening form. It therefore "protected" her from being consumed by overwhelming, debilitating anxiety. So rather than explore the meaning and relevance of her nightmare, I decided on a safer, less precarious approach. We would explore her daytime fantasy of the barn from the week before. My hope was that both paths would lead to the same place.

But first I needed to acknowledge her nightmare. "That's a very scary dream. You must have been terrified."

Sue nodded.

Then I continued: "I've been thinking of another possibly scary experience that you mentioned last time. You remembered standing in a dark barn as a kid looking out at the rectangle of light representing the outside world."

"Yeah, I used to do that a lot. But no one knew about it."

"Did you want someone to know?"

"Well, like I said last time, it felt lonely."

Her loneliness and isolation were the toxins to her developing sense of self—the conditions that had threatened her with an imminent symbolic death.

"And from whom did you feel most disconnected?" I asked.

"My mother." Sue took all of one nanosecond to answer.

It was time to resume what we had started last week. This time I asked Sue to stand up and again put her imaginary mother in the chair. I then beckoned her to play act both roles of a dialogue with her mother about the rectangle of light, specifically one that she *wished* had occurred so many years ago.

Sue   "Mom, do you know that I spend hours and hours in the dark barn?"

Mom   [I motion for Sue to sit in the empty chair and become her Mom] "No, I didn't know that. What's wrong? Please tell me!"

Sue   "Remember when you asked me if I heard the birds singing outside? I said 'yes.' But I couldn't hear them. I can't hear them. You know how we all laugh at the comedians on Ed Sullivan? I can never hear them either! Remember when you asked me if I liked school. I hate school! I hate school! I can't do it! Everyone expects me to be normal. I'm not! I'm hard-of-hearing. I'm not a bad person, I'm not a stupid person, I'm just hard-of-hearing!"

By this time, Sue was yelling and beating the pillow which she had placed on her lap. I then asked her to become her mother again.

Thrpst   [to Sue] "Do you understand your daughter's pain?"

Mom   [sullen] "Yes, I do."

Thrpst   "Would you tell her about it?"

Mom   [looks at empty chair] "Sue, I've tried so hard to act like everything's all right. To protect you from the pain. From my pain. To act like there's nothing to worry about. Like you can do it. You just don't know how many nights your Dad and I stay up worrying about you, trying to figure out—"

Sue   [switches seats herself] "You never told me that, Mom."

Mom   [switches seats] "It has been really tough for you to have a hearing loss. I know that. You've had to pretend so much, bluffing your way through life. If I only had known! If I only had known that you hid from people, hid from us, even hid from yourself. If I only had known the shame you felt. I would have held you and made it all better if I could."

Thrpst "You can't take away her being hard-of-hearing, but you can still help. Would you tell Sue how you can make it better for her?"

Mom "Sue, you don't have normal hearing, that's a fact. That means you cannot do certain things; you have some limitations. But it doesn't mean you're stupid or defective. It means having to continually educate resistant people of what it means to be hard-of-hearing—people like teachers, coworkers, and even therapists. It means feeling frustrated while trying to figure out what you can do and accepting what you can't do. Being hard-of-hearing means all of those things. I'm so sorry I didn't help you openly acknowledge all of this with me. I'm sorry. I've come to realize that it's okay that you, or anyone for that matter, can't do certain things. It's okay. We are still competent. We are still good people, God's children. [with tears] I love you, you know."

Sue [to Mom] "You're not perfect. That's okay. Better late than never. [with tears] I love you, too."

The enacted dialogue temporarily reached a comfortable resting point. For several minutes, Sue and I sat still in our seats, taking in all that had happened. Sue was clearly beginning to work through the pain of feeling let down and emotionally abandoned by her mother. Her fear and rage had given way to longing and sadness.

But our work was not done. It would have been both unfair and unhealthy for us to have portrayed Sue only as a victim of her "big, bad," neglectful mother. So-called "mother-bashing" is a frequent but false path. It is very tempting to forget that Sue's mother, too, was a victim of society's denial of disabilities. The predominant medical model had taught Sue and her parents early on to implicitly shield the other from what seemed to them the overwhelming pain of managing hearing loss. They would discuss only sterile medical information and medical management in a perfunctory and superficial manner. However, in contrast to making the effects of hearing loss go away or even reaping certain benefits, their tacit agreement to shield each other made everything worse.

Unfortunately, as with many persons with acquired hearing loss, this dysfunctional arrangement was not limited to Sue's family. It was significant that Sue through role playing her mother intimated that she even had to convince psychotherapists of the psychological challenges of hearing loss. She had previously received psychotherapy for two years from a therapist who, like her parents, had denied all of these effects. Sue complained that she spent many sessions trying to describe how it felt to have a hearing loss. "My therapist diagnosed me as being histrionic, as rationalizing my problems, and as having a personality disorder. And when I got angry at her, she accused me of transferring my anger at my parents onto her! It felt like she was blaming me!"

Sue was not acting out her unresolved anger with that therapist, but was in actuality being retraumatized by her. Like Sue's parents, many therapists are not sufficiently informed of the psychological ramifications of acquired hearing loss. Many are also overanxious about not knowing how to be with such clients and end up colluding with the client's family in their denial. Sue's previous therapist, inasmuch as she was not competent to treat persons with hearing loss, was also unethical in her denial.

After approximately one year, my sessions with Sue were coming to an end. We had met biweekly, sometimes once a month, in total about twenty visits. Sue and I had walked through grief's center together, through the pain and emotional resolution of the fragmented relationship with her parents, particularly her mother. Toward the end of treatment, I asked Sue to write a letter to her parents that she may never send and to imagine what she would want her parents to write back. This is a common ritual to help adults recover from the effects of childhood trauma.[5] What follows are segments from both letters.

From Sue to her parents.

Dear Mom and Dad,

I hope all is well with you, and that daddy's back feels better. It has taken me a long time to write this letter, about forty years, because I was afraid you'd be mad or hurt for what I have to tell you. But I can't—or rather don't want to—hold my feelings in and hide myself from you anymore. That has taken too much of a toll on my life.

You really don't know me, and you never have. If you only had known the pain I have carried around inside of me, even as a kid. Instead, you saw a little girl with pigtails who loved Turkish taffy, who played on the jungle gym, and who loved blowing bubbles. If only you had known that the little girl had no idea of where she ended and others began. If only you had known how much I had tried to please you and daddy, by doing well at school, by not going to my bedroom every Thanksgiving and Christmas to escape all those people, and by eating at the dinner table, nodding my head or smiling at strategic points in the conversation in order to pretend that I could follow it.

Please don't blame all this on my ears, cuz it's not that simple. If I had no legs, you wouldn't force me to jump! If I was blind, you wouldn't force me to drive a car. So why did you force me to hear when I couldn't?

Finally now at age forty-one, I know that my pain and my feeling that I had failed you and me (and for that matter, everyone else) WASN'T MY FAULT. If only you had known to tell me that; if only you had known to tell yourselves that. If only you had been told. If only. . . .

I love you, Sue

Sue's imagined letter from her parents.

Dear Sue,

I can't remember how many nights, after you had gone to bed, your father and I cried for you. I still see you walking by yourself in crowds, looking so cut off from the world. I would tell everyone during family gatherings, and even during dinner, to speak slowly and clearly (particularly Uncle George who always mumbled) but it was no good. They wouldn't listen. How ironic that I expected you to listen when all those hearing people couldn't.

You now know that I am not as tall or as smart or as sensitive or as good as you had hoped and had assumed. And I dare say, I now know that myself. I'm so so sorry! The truth is that your hearing loss was so painful to me (and daddy) that I pretended you were fine; and, I guess, we also made you pretend you were fine.

No, I'm not hurt or angry at you for your letter. It took a lot of guts for you to write it! Oh how I wish we could have been able to talk like this when you had pigtails and kept getting Turkish taffy stuck in your braces (remember that?). If I only could have not hid my helplessness and pain from you, and from daddy. Maybe I wouldn't have been so alone, too! I could have hugged you, dear, and cried with you, and afterward could have made you that meatball dish that you liked so much.

The pain, rage, and denial that we both fell victim to wasn't because of your ears. If only I had known not to let your hearing loss pollute your life and mine. It didn't have to. If only I had known what to do. If only someone had told me. I'm sorry.

I love you.

Love, Mom and Dad.

As Sue read these letters to me, we both became teary. To this day, I cannot read her letters aloud without welling up. Her search for validation touches a deep part of me as well.

After a few more meetings, Sue felt that it was time to say goodbye. "Maybe not forever," she added, "but for now." Parting felt right to me as well. Sue had bravely reopened old wounds that had never sufficient healed. She began a healing process that both of us had not realized was awaiting our attention. From then on, those inevitable "problems in living" that originally had brought her into treatment would no longer become debilitating liabilities. We bid each other good luck and farewell.

That was a year ago. One night, as I was writing this chapter, Sue coincidentally left a message on my answering machine to return her call as soon as possible. I telephoned her immediately. She told me that her mother had passed away. It had been several months prior and peacefully in her sleep.

"Before she died," Sue reported, "we talked about the good and bad parts of my growing up. Afterward, we hugged and said we loved each other. The next morning, my Mom was gone."

I said how sorry I was, but how lucky both of them were to have made that opportunity to say goodbye.

"But that is not why I called," she quickly emphasized. Apparently, Sue and her Dad were rummaging through the attic and found her mother's diary. Sue wanted to read to me a particularly relevant passage:

Dear Diary,

Today we had Sue's fifth birthday party and I just finished baking her a chocolate cake. It has been three months since the audiologist confirmed her hearing loss. But until last week, we thought it would not affect her much. We thanked God we lived in a beautiful neighborhood with plenty of kids her age and a child community center.

Last Monday, a group of kids were in the playground and they invited Sue to join them. Her exuberance and joy for being included was unforgettable. But then, while she was climbing on the jungle gym, the children ran to the backyard to play hide-and-go-seek. When Sue turned around, she wondered what had happened. She cried. It seemed a foreboding of things to come that I found unbearable. Right at that moment, I whisked her up in my arms and carried her home where she wouldn't be alone.

At home, we played our own games—Chutes and Ladders and Checkers. Anything to make her forget about it. She never mentioned that incident and got happy again.

———

In summarizing a therapeutic odyssey, it is tempting to highlight only the magic moments when everything seems to click and not to emphasize the less dramatic stretches of time. Because of the brevity of this story, I, too, am guilty of such selective reporting. Consequently, the reader may erroneously get the impression that Sue and I skipped along a primrose path with enlightenments at every corner. In the words of Alfred Hitchcock, "Drama is life with the dull bits cut out."

When I think of Sue, I find myself most impressed not so much with the dramatic moments of our work together, but with her earnestness and tenacity. Sue was not a quitter! And neither were her parents. Both met their challenges head on with the best information available at the time. But I shared Sue's sadness about what feelings had never been shared until her mother was on her deathbed.

If only they had known.

Notes

1. Wolf, E. S. (1988). *Treating the self: Elements of clinical self psychology.* New York: Guilford Press.

2. Hamilton, N. G. (1988). *Self and others: Object relations theory in practice.* Northvale, NJ: Jason Aronson, Inc.

3. Kohut, H. (1971). *The analysis of the self.* New York: International Universities Press.

4. Rigsby, J. (1991). *My grieving heart.* Hagerstown, MD: Autumn House Publishing Co.

5. Bass, E., & Davis, L. (1988). *The courage to heal: A guide for women survivors of child sexual abuse.* New York: Harper & Row.

CHAPTER THREE

Progressive Hearing Loss, Men, and Our Fathers

What was immediately striking about Steven was his tough-looking, gruff exterior. He looked much older than his thirty-eight years, with prominent, inlaid lines in his forehead as a testimony to his hard life. His wife had referred him for individual psychotherapy. She felt that he had become cantankerous due to the fertility difficulties they were having and his hearing loss. She adamantly refused to participate in couples therapy, insisting that it was *his* problem. So Steven begrudgingly came to see me by himself, and made a point of informing me that "just for the record" he was being "dragged to a shrink" by his wife.

On entering my office for our first session, Steven carried a thick, leather file folder containing a collection of meticulously organized medical, psychological, and audiological evaluations. Before I could formally invite him to begin our dialogue, he methodically presented all of the audiograms that had been done since he was nineteen years old. At that time, his hearing loss was described as "mild, but with excellent speech discrimination."

As Steven read through the documented indictments of how his loss has progressed to severe/profound with poor speech discrimination, his demeanor changed from gruff-ness to detachment and his words became more scientific and devoid of emotion. He elucidated the implications of pure tone thresholds, recruitment, the speech frequency range, and other audiological principles. It felt like he was giving me a lecture with a final exam around the corner.

Twenty minutes had slowly passed. "You know this mate-rial quite well," I finally interjected.

"I should, I've lived through it, haven't I?" He scowled, looked at his watch, and promptly resumed the lesson. So much for my attempt to connect with him. I had failed the first test.

Steven's didactics then proceeded to cover the techno-logical aspects of air/bone conduction and auditory thresh-olds, then recruitment, and then basilar membrane tissue. He ended the lesson by listing all the incompetent audiolo-gists he had met.

"You've had a lot of unhelpful assistance." Attempt num-ber two.

"Doc, you have no idea what hard-of-hearing people have to go through. No idea. Zilch! You doctors hide be-hind those fancy degrees of yours and just pretend to know how to help. You sit there in your fancy offices, in your fancy buildings, with your fancy equipment, and with your fancy fees, but you don't know what the hell you're talking about; what it's like on the other side; how insensitive the world is and how many things you hearing people take for granted." He paused, looked me over a bit, and gave me a parting jab. "And you don't have to get so defensive on me!"

Me, defensive? How could he know that? My facial expres-sion? My posture? Although I knew that his pain fueled his offense, he nevertheless made me feel like an incompetent member of the hearing, enemy team. Despite my well-in-grained understanding that one does not have the power to make another person feel anything, I felt threatened by Steven.

Steven was right about one thing. When it came to understanding his experience, I became a student—one who was full of curiosity and interest. I needed to concur with Steven about knowing nothing about the psychological effects of his loss and invite him to educate me—to teach me what his hearing loss meant to him. At some point, I would need to acknowledge his distress, but not now. It was too early in our relationship.

"I have no idea how you experience your hearing loss," I said half-meekly, half-confidently. "I hope that you can teach me."

He reluctantly nodded his head and agreed to a second appointment.

Steven was straight out of a male psychology book, a man who tried to be a "real man" the only way he knew how—to be gruff, strong, and distant. His father, consumed with the same challenge, did as his father had taught him. He worked fourteen-hour days and made lots of money. He too was gruff, strong, and distant.

As the oldest of two children, Steven had excelled at whatever he did. He made the high school varsity team in basketball, football, and soccer. He starred in two drama productions, was on the debate team, and played the saxophone in the school band. He feigned annoyance about having to help his younger brother with math homework, but was secretly flattered. Steven knew his parents were proud of him.

In times of victory, Steven shared with his mother how it felt to win and be "the best." For his father, Steven displayed rows of his trophies with the hope that he would notice them, and sure enough, within hours of each addition, his dad would give him a high five and tell him to "keep it up."

It remained like this for years. For some reason, in his junior year, Steven slowly began to lose his edge. He messed up on a couple of key basketball plays, causing his team to lose an important game, which was very atypical for him. His general performance became a bit sporadic. During drama rehearsals, he began to "daydream too much," which prompted the director to tell him once again to pay attention. He also began to mope at home.

After a while, his mother would half-derisively and half-affectionately chide him for being in his own world— "you're just like your dad." His father had a different view. At this juncture, he took his cue to get more directly involved in coaching his son. "You got to make the grade! Being second best is being a loser. C'mon you can do it!" His dad even began to show up at sports matches.

"There's nothing that you can't do if you put your mind to it."

Those words became his father's ritualistic slogan, and, in turn, those words would continually echo in Steven's mind as his guiding mantra. When he couldn't do something, he tried harder; he put his mind to it.

His father's teachings had strong precedent as part of the American Dream: the Horatio Algiers story that anyone can succeed by expending enough effort; our country's underdog victory against the British to gain our independence, about which we were endlessly taught in grade school. In a well-known children's book, the train almost couldn't make it up the hill until it tried harder. "Karate Kid." "Rocky." We expect ourselves to be able to jump tall buildings with a single bound if we try hard enough.

In this manner, Steven went all out to make the grade, to lead his team in points scored, to earn the respect and admiration of the drama director, his teachers, other students and, most of all, his mom and dad. He got mercilessly angry and down on himself when he failed to pay attention and when he screwed up. This led to more work, more practice, and more discipline. There's nothing that you can't do if you put your mind to it. More practice. More losing his edge. More practice. More screw ups. More practice. More screw ups.

Somewhere amidst this cycle of defeats, Steven insidiously began to experience shame. That was new. Shame had never been part of Steven's repertoire. He knew only vaguely about the concept from his introduction to psychology class—it was included on a quiz that he had not studied for. He did recall thinking that shame applied to other people, probably to his sister, who constantly cried about something or other, or to "boy sissies."

Shame is "metastasized" guilt. Steven had experienced repeated guilt as a result of many, in his words, "screw ups"—"if only I could have gotten my act together to do. . . ." As his individual frustrations and failures continued to multiply, they soon became the norm rather than the exception. Guilt about his poor performances had "metastasized"— had generalized—to become shame about his whole sense of self.

Shame was not part of his father's repertoire either. By this time, his ritual pep talks took on more of the flavor of beratements: "no son of mine is going to be a sissy and give up, so stop your whining and. . . ." Steven's mother, in turn, chided his father: "Now, dear, don't you think you're being too hard on Steven?" They fought. As the family alliances formed with his mother tentatively comforting Steven, his father felt he had to prevent him from becoming a "mamma's boy." So he berated Steven even more. Soon his beratements became verbal, emotional abuse.

It is a sad but familiar story how a lot of unnecessary psychological damage is done to children with acquired hearing loss before the loss is identified. During the prediagnosis stage, Steven's hearing loss had already become woven into the fabric of the family drama. His guilt and shame were now embedded in the structure of the family's alliances, conflicts, and models of what it meant to be a man.

Since Steven was unable to stand up to his father and unable to understand his mother's tentative support coupled with her helpless withdrawal, he retreated behind a wall of loneliness and pain that even he did not consciously acknowledge. Behind that wall, he was immersed in the anguish that he had incorporated from his dad's own defective sense of self and shame that had never been worked through.

During our sessions, however, Steven expressed rage as a substitute for his walled-in pain. He berated me as his father had berated him. "Now listen to me will you, doc! You don't know what the hell you're talking about!" He would scream at me, wave his fist in the air, and pound his fist on the seat. His face once became so red that I was scared he would have a coronary right there.

During one episode, I wondered if he was about to assault me. I felt my eyes carefully look toward the door, mapping out an emergency exit plan.

"Why the hell am I coming to see you anyway? Why? Why? I don't need this! Why am I here? Huh? You goddamn doctors; I'm sick of all of you. . . ." For the time being, his assaults on me were only verbal.

I was about to verbally assault him back with his own question: "Yeah, why are you coming to see me anyway? Huh? Huh?" But in the middle of that fantasy, discipline overpowered my insecurities. No. Returning his assault would not have been helpful, and it might have fueled his fire.

Not knowing what else to do, I simply remained seated with him. I waited.

Seeing no offensive reaction from me, he softened a bit. His face changed from beet red to only dark pink, and his voice became a bit slower. After a pause, he continued: "You and other people need to stop your self-righteous arrogance and stop feeling sorry for hearing-impaired people. We can do anything that you can."

His veneer of rage was beginning to crack and to expose his pain. In response to Steven, I took care to make my voice softer and slower, although inside I was still a bit shaken. The awesome power of another's soul never ceases to humble me.

I paused. "You said earlier that hearing people take things for granted. Would you tell me what you mean?"

"Now, that's a good question," Steven eagerly retorted.

Steven regained his composure from his previous outburst. On familiar ground again, he responded as my teacher, and I, once again, became his student. It was comfortable like before, but I could not help wondering whether I inadvertently distracted him from his pain for my own comfort? In looking back, I think his torment scared me more than I had realized.

Familiar scenarios. The seemingly thousands of times he had telephoned employment possibilities, only to ask them repeatedly what they were saying; no jobs; high-frequency sounds; telephone answering machines; conversations beyond his range of speech discrimination; parties, bars, and restaurants where he became isolated among crowds of people. Inasmuch as Steven blamed the world for not taking him seriously, on a more personal level, he blamed himself for his demise. Shame was the price he paid for his steadfast loyalty to his father: "There's nothing that you can't do if you put your mind to it."

Steven continued his stories. But instead of anguish, his words became more filled with pedagogy. "You know, Dr. Harvey, the world needs to know that hearing impaired people appear to understand more than they do. I can't tell you how many times I've been to meetings at work during which the boss would get up and give an important talk and a discussion would happen. I would again and again have to tell them to get an audio loop. You know, an audio loop is. . . . And you know about the ADA [American Disabilities

Act], don't you? I would threaten to report them and to hire an attorney to guarantee that I get equal accessibility. And furthermore, people need to understand that. . . ."

He continued for a half-hour. A familiar cycle. Pedagogy, anger, more pedagogy. How do I intervene?

Meekly, I commented that coping with the hearing world must have felt frustrating.

"What does frustration have to do with it? Do you understand that this is a matter of civil rights? Do you understand that. . . ?" His voice got louder and his face redder.

Here we go again. By this time, I had become familiar with the symptoms of Steven's pain, as manifested by his anger: namely, the tightness in *my* stomach and the gnawing self-depreciation of *my* thoughts. Unable to integrate or tolerate his pain, he denied it, projected it onto me, and lectured me until I felt his pain as my own. Technically this is called projective identification.[1] It is also exemplified by a cartoon of a couple on an airplane. One spouse asks the other, "do you want to be scared on this trip or should I?"

Steven had mastered the skill of "giving his pain to someone else to hold" from his father. His dad had internalized Steven's decline in performance as a severe blow to his own self esteem, perhaps thinking at some level that he had failed in his parenting. By continually drilling into Steven that "There's nothing that you can't do if you put your mind to it," he absolved himself of blame. It was Steven, not himself, who was not trying hard enough, who was "wimping out." Steven came to feel what had begun as his father's shame and low self-esteem.

Similarly, during the therapy hour, I felt Steven's shame as my own. By continually putting me in my place with his academic and technical assaults, he was unconsciously giving me his self-depreciatory feelings to hold. I often felt anxious and doubtful of my therapeutic abilities. In this manner, Steven could spare himself that emotional burden.

I began to become irritated but kept this emerging feeling private.

Just as I hoped his tutorial would end and we could talk about emotional issues or at least have a dialogue, he produced a copy of an article I had written entitled "Between Two Worlds: One Psychologist's View of the Hard-of-Hearing Experience."[2] He began to wave it in front of me.

"Oh, shit!" I thought to myself.

"I have several criticisms of what you wrote, doctor!"

I did not miss his "doctor" sarcasm, but I knew better than to attempt an interpretation, namely, that he was zapping me to avoid looking at some painful issues about himself. Admittedly, I was stunned and probably a bit defensive once again. So I sat silently.

"I'm IN the hearing world, not out of it, like you suggest. And here, on page four you say, 'The usual reactions [to missing oral communication] are to cover up, minimize, deny, overcompensate. . . .'" That's pure hogwash! I insist on understanding what people are saying. How could you imply that. . . ."

He continued for the remaining minutes of our session. It was finally time to stop. We had gone nowhere. "Maybe I had some Tylenol in my desk," I thought to myself. If not, I would surely have to stop at the drug store.

As Steven stood up to leave—perhaps as a way of softening his assaults on me—he mentioned that he had a lot of errands to do. His dad's retirement party was planned for the next weekend. It would be a formal event at a nearby country club with over 100 friends and family members. I commented that it sounded like it would be fun and wished him success on his errands. We exchanged goodbyes.

A week later, his wife left a message on my answering machine, saying that Steven was sick and could not make our scheduled appointment. I found myself frankly both relieved and upset that this perhaps meant that he was leaving therapy. No more lectures. I wondered if he had sensed my impatience or irritation? What else I could have done to forge an emotional—as opposed to didactic—connection with him? What had I done wrong?

Steven did come back the following week, on time as usual; however he looked uncharacteristically disheveled and somewhat pale. I noticed the scraggly beginnings of a beard: he had not shaven for at least several days. In answer to my looks of concern, he told me that he had been bedridden for over a week with pleurisy, a painful lung ailment, accompanied by a fever of over 104 degrees! For the most part, he had been unable to even lift his head off the pillow.

Steven had missed his dad's party.

The triumph of mind over body is assured until your body is real sick. Most of us have had the humbling experience of trying harder to get out of bed, only to find that our body will not allow it.

I said in earnest how sorry I was, to which he replied, "Thanks, doc. Shit happens."

"Yes it does," I agreed. We shared a real moment that I did not want to spoil, but it seemed like an important and rare therapeutic opportunity, so I broke the awkward silence: "But why didn't you just try harder?" I consciously raised my eyebrows to accentuate the intent of my question as playful but provocative.

"Stuff it doc, will ya!" was his knee-jerk reply.

"C'mon Steven. I don't get it. "There's nothing that you can't do if you put your mind to it."

"Shut up!" he yelled.

"There's nothing you can't do if—"

"Shut up!" he yelled. "Enough! I get your point! NOW SHUT UP WITH THIS, WILL YA?"

This time I did shut up. Now in a soft voice, I said to Steven, "Listen, I want you to know that I'm really sorry you couldn't make the party. I know how much it must have meant to you."

Steven muttered "thanks."

Although I could not know what missing his dad's party meant to him, my intent was to convey compassion, particularly on the heels of what he could have understandably perceived as my "rubbing salt in his wounds." I did not wish to be cruel or insensitive, but it seemed critically important for me to somehow challenge his steadfast belief that he could do the impossible if only he tried hard enough, a belief that had caused him much guilt and shame.

In a limited sense, getting out of bed with pleurisy can be compared to comprehending many muffled, oral conversations with a significant hearing loss. You cannot overcome either obstacle by "putting your mind to it." No matter how much Steven would try, he inevitably felt conversationally lost in noisy, oral group situations in which hearing persons simultaneously vollied for attention.

"Sometimes those who put their minds to it and try and try again do in fact fail," I offered, this time in a gentle voice.

"I've been investigating cochlear implants. You probably don't know that they have. . . ."

Rather than question his father's teachings, Steven had abruptly changed the subject. His next tutorial had begun. Instead of succumbing to his psychological defense of pedagogy as I had done before by waiting until his lecture ended, I decided to more directly confront his steadfast loyalty to his father. It was this rigidified loyalty to "There's nothing that you can't do if you put your mind to it" that kept Steven stuck in a never-ending cycle of shame and rage. If I could help him get unstuck, I surmised that maybe I could then get Steven to comfort and sooth himself more.

"Excuse me," I interrupted. "What did your dad teach you about how to manage your hearing loss?" This time *I* abruptly changed the subject.

"My dad was a fighter!" he instantly replied.

"I know that, but how did he help you manage your hearing loss?"

"He taught me not to give up."

"Has it worked?"

"You're damn right it has," Steven scowled.

"Then why are you here?" I retorted.

"I told you five weeks ago. My wife wouldn't get off my back if I didn't come and. . . ."

"But Steven, that was the first time. Maybe the second. But you keep coming. You're on time every meeting. You're prepared every meeting. You come every week. You must come for a reason."

"I come, that's why!" he scowled.

"You must have a reason. Nobody's forcing you to come now. C'mon. Why? Why?" By this time, I was raising my voice.

After an awkward pause Steven looked down toward the floor, out the window, and then at the door. He stuttered a bit, saying something I could not decipher. He was clearly thrown off balance. I watched him stammer as he tried to think of what to say. Instead he remained speechless. I had him in checkmate.

Now I needed to pause, not to observe Steven but to observe myself. How did our dialogue—an intimate, psychological odyssey—degenerate into a competition, a chess game; two men having a jousting match? (There is a sexist joke that goes "How many men does it take to screw in a light bulb? It doesn't matter. They'll fight over who goes first.")

It was not difficult to figure out why things went wrong. This jostling had an all too familiar quality to it. As a child, I had always tried to please my own dad, typically by beating him at board games. My belief was that beating my dad would somehow initiate me into the grownup world; it would have made me a man. However, he always beat me at whatever game we played. I could never win!

With Steven, however, I was beginning to "win." I recalled how, during our first appointment, he somehow got under my skin. He came out fighting and I struggled to defend myself. At an unconscious level, I guess I was afraid that he would beat me just like my dad. I was afraid Steven would turn me into a little boy.

For each of us, our dialogue was experienced as a repetition of our earlier competition with our fathers.

It is impossible for therapists to prevent such intrusions from their own pasts. They inevitably and often quite insidiously intercede in treatment. Rather, the task is to recognize the effects of one's own emotional vulnerabilities, to analyze their origins, and to prevent them from polluting the therapeutic interaction.

My triumphant glee coupled with shock and guilt were red flags that I was reacting to Steven as if he were someone else. My excursion backward in time to my family of origin was quite brief, lasting only a few blinks, for it is a familiar journey. I frequently revisit old conversations with my dad.

During these "few blinks," Steven shuffled a bit in his chair, seemingly about to surrender or plan a counterattack. He sensed my glee but not its resolution. Having recovered from acting-out my own issues, now my task was to find a way to help him question the adequacy of how his father had coped with a favorite son who had a hearing loss.

"Maybe you could sort of walk me through how you would help your son or daughter if he or she acquired a hearing loss," I finally said.

"I don't have a son."

"What if you do? You're going for a fertility workup, I know. What if he, assuming it's a boy, becomes deaf or hard-of-hearing?"

Steven squirmed in his seat, again looked out the window for a bit, and then positioned his eyes toward the floor. This time, however, I felt compassion for his pain. My own father, at least for now, was no longer "in the room." Steven breathed more slowly and looked up at me. In a soft and solemn voice, he confidently made an affirmation: "I would tell my son to come to me when he's down. I'd be there for him; I'd listen." His words echoed from his soul.

A couple of seconds passed. Perhaps to ensure that the safety of his old self was still there, he quickly added "But not so much that I'd make him a wimp!"

"God forbid, be careful of that!" I quipped. We exchanged a glance.

Steven knew it was now safe. So he continued, this time in a low, tender voice: "I'd be there for him, you know? I would tell him that I care and that I love him. And that you don't have to be afraid to show your fears, your weaknesses, your anger, your frustration, the things you so quickly push out of your mind. You don't need to hide all that from me. I'm your dad. And I love you."

He paused and closed his eyes. Slowly and softly he gave his future son the gift that he now knew his father had never been able to give him: "I'm your dad. We'll get through this together. You don't have to be ashamed with me."

For the first time, I saw Steven's tears. And for the first time, he saw mine.

He continued, his voice remaining soft and solemn. "You know, my dad and I camped together, ran together, drank beers together. He took me to my first Red Sox game—I was only five years old! I remember when he gave me his old hunting knife, it was all rusty, dirty. I still have it."

"I bet you do. What do you think he was saying to you by giving you his knife."

"It was a goddamn knife, doc, that's all. Quit interpreting every goddamn thing, will ya?" He half scowled, half grinned. An abrupt shift.

"It's a professional liability. I'm terribly sorry." We exchanged a smile.

Steven sat quiet and still. And soon, more tears came. "We never stopped doing things together, you know? But after I lost my hearing we never again looked each other straight in the eyes. I not only lost my hearing, I lost my dad, too." He paused. "I wish he hadn't left."

We fell silent for several moments.

"You'll be a good father, Steven."

He looked at me somewhat inquisitively amidst tears and then slowly nodded his head.

As it was already past time for us to stop, it was me, for a change, who motioned to end our meeting. We already had a next appointment. Upon leaving, Steven bid me to "take care."

Although our next meeting contained more glimmers of his pain and anguish, it was as if he had opened the window into his soul too wide and too quickly, and now he had to slam it shut. That session and the ones to follow once again came to resemble tutorials. Steven instructed me about the bio-psycho-social ramifications of hearing loss as he had done in the beginning of our relationship. He also told me about his latest research on getting a cochlear implant.

One day, he began our meeting by announcing "my wife says I don't have to come anymore." Although he admitted that she noticed that he had become more content and at peace, Steven himself denied any internal changes. We had met for eleven sessions over a period of six months.

Our termination was bittersweet. To this day, I relish the softening in Steven that I observed, our largely unspoken closeness, and how he had touched my own pain. I also lament that we could not talk more openly and directly about his anguish, and that his "window" could not have remained open longer. When I think of Steven, I recall a quotation by Henry Thoreau: "The mass of men live lives of quiet desperation." At these times, I also often think of my Dad.

Around the time when my work with Steven ended, my father challenged me to yet one more game of chess. I complied, once again preparing myself to handle defeat. After all, at that time I was only a thirty-eight-year-old "kid." But I won! In fact, I won easily. That victory, too, was bittersweet. For I realized that although beating him in chess symbolized my entry into competent adulthood, my victory also symbolized my loss of idealizing him as a divine sort of mentor and comforter, and as a shield protecting me from facing my own eventual death. In a way, I wish I could have replayed that chess game. With both Steven and my father, I relearned that winning isn't everything.

It was obvious that Steven did not quite know how to say goodbye to me. I had just finished telling him how much I appreciated and was touched by the work he had done. As had happened many times before, here again his "window" opened and then shut. His voice became soft, as he said "thank you, doc, thank you for everything." He shook my hand. I returned his shake and clasped his hand with both of mine. We looked each other straight in the eye and then his voice abruptly reverted back to a didactic mode. He advised me, "Don't forget what I've taught you." But then he smiled and gave me further advice: "Maybe you should write about this so others can read it."

"Good idea. Maybe I will."

Three years later, I received an announcement from Steven and his wife. They had a baby boy, 8 lbs, 3 oz. I knew that Steven would be a good father.

Notes

1. Ogden, T. H. (1979). On projective identification. *International Journal of Psycho-Analysis,* 60, 357–373.
2. Harvey, M. A. (1985). Between two worlds: One psychologist's view of the hard-of-hearing person's experience. *SHHH,* 6(4), 4–5.

CHAPTER FOUR

Changing the Rules of Trival Pursuit

Only minutes after introducing himself, Robert told me about a recurring nightmare that he had been having for over a decade: "I'm leaving my house when suddenly the whole world becomes a Trivial Pursuit board. Everybody I meet becomes a Trivial Pursuit card. A voice tells me that I'm gonna die unless I answer the questions on all of the cards correctly. I'm terrified because I don't know enough to do that. Then I scream and wake up in a cold sweat."

He first experienced these nighttime excursions of terror as an adolescent, several years after sustaining a severe hearing loss at the age of four, presumably as a result of a high fever. Over the past several years, his hearing slowly deteriorated to profound deafness. He was now thirty-five years old.

In discussing the significance of his nightmares, he recalled feeling similarly terrified in elementary school when he was asked to play games such as Concentration, Jeopardy, or Hollywood Squares. "First of all," he reported, "even if I could understand the teacher, which was iffy at best, I usually couldn't understand the other kids. Second, I usually didn't know the answers. All the kids would laugh at me."

Although Robert was above average in intelligence, unfortunately there were no accommodations made in his home and mainstream school environments which would have increased his opportunities to incidentally "pick up" information. At school, there were no consistent support services, such as assistive listening devices, sign language, oral interpretation, or preferential seating. At home, he appeared to understand everything but understood little.

His memories of games like Jeopardy and Trivial Pursuit, which measured so-called incidental learning, functioned as metaphors for how he felt in the world: inadequate and terrified. Neither his waking hours nor his sleep provided respite.

It took Robert well over half of our meeting to explain his nightmare and associations to it and still I had no idea why he opted to begin psychotherapy now.

"That's easy," he began. "For a long time, I haven't dated anyone. But now some woman at work wants to go out with me. She's really attractive and super smart. I'm afraid I'll make a fool of myself." He sat stiffly in his seat, seemingly holding on for dear life, as he continued to explain what seemed like a variation on the Trivial Pursuit theme.

"My hearing impairment is a constant cloud hanging over me which prevents me from achieving any success or getting too close to people. I get scared that I don't know enough or that I'll make a fool of myself and that people will laugh at me. It's easier to stay home!"

He avoided making eye contact with me, instead looking down at the floor or squirming in his seat. I imagined Robert's view of himself as one massive dark, dense, "hearing-impairment" cloud full of failure, misery, anxiety, and torment. What does one do with such a cloud? Is there anything else? I fantasized about searching for some sun, blue sky, or any other scenery that his cloud might be hiding.

I asked him to tell me another part of his story: "Are you sure it's your 'hearing impairment'—the cloud—that's keeping you stuck? Nothing's that simple."

My question was an initial challenge for Robert to stop oversimplifying his difficulty and acknowledge its complexity. For starters, he would need to separate his disability from his handicaps.

A disability is an objectively measurable medical condition. What I am calling an external handicap refers to the obstacles that the environment places on a person with a disability. For example, if there are no curb cuts, wheelchair users cannot access the sidewalk. If there is no communication access, deaf users cannot understand what people are saying. There are also internal handicaps. What begin as obstacles in one's environment (external handicaps) eventually become internalized as emotional obstacles to achieving healthy self-esteem and psychological growth.

A description of Robert's disability was clear. He had a bilateral, sensorineural, severe-to-profound hearing loss, with no measurable hearing above 2K Hz. His unaided speech discrimination score was zero. We can graph his hearing loss on an audiogram, quantify it with aided versus unaided scores, measure the amount of reflex decay, and chart the peak latencies of his auditory brainstem response.

A description of his external handicaps was already given: namely, a history of limited accommodations and support services in his home and school. These handicaps prevented him from receiving environmental information which is normally transmitted on three overlapping levels:[1]

1. the language level: written or verbal information exchange. For example, formal or information conversations.

2. the warning level: signals of potentially dangerous events. For example, sirens, thunder, and car horns beeping.

3. the primitive level: loosely described as the auditory "rumble" of daily living which "connects" us to our surroundings. The sound of the wind, crickets, and birds.

A description of his internal handicaps, however, was more complex. "It's a strange thing," Robert began. "I feel cut off from the world in so many ways. As I said before, it's like a cloud." Because of a long history of feeling frustrated by inadequate environmental accommodations, he learned to feel ill-equipped and inferior. Instead of blaming the environment for creating his handicapping situation, he eventually succumbed to blaming himself. He had been psychologically battered into viewing most situations as critical tests of his competence.

Therefore, a chance meeting with a friend at a beach (where he did not wear hearing aids) petrified him—"what if I don't understand what she's saying? That will mean I'm dumb." Any group or social gathering—typically in dark, noisy restaurants and bars—elicited similar anxiety. In terms of his self-esteem, he had commented to me that he sometimes felt "two inches tall, like I have no right taking up space on this earth." His negative "self-talk" and withdrawal even generalized to one-to-one situations in which he could have easily functioned. With me, he often did not make eye contact, was dressed in wrinkled, unkempt clothes, and looked much older than his age of thirty-five.

His previous disability of severe hearing loss and now his profound deafness were not only self evident, but also presented real and inevitable challenges. To deny their impact was counterproductive.

External handicaps also, by definition, create obstacles, but they do not have to. All too often, however, the disabled person does not attempt to remove those external handicaps. It is typically not because of laziness or lack of ability. Rather, I have found that persons with hearing loss too frequently accept a wide array of internal handicapping self-depreciatory beliefs as self-evident truths which are beyond scrutiny. Often one cannot remove external handicaps until one deals with the internal handicapping beliefs.

It would be important to show Robert that he could choose another belief system and that there were options for how he could view himself and his world other than those he knew at present. It is our ability to construct our own reality that distinguishes us as humans. In fact, psychotherapy can be defined as "an interpersonal agreement to abrogate the usual rules that structure reality in order to reshape reality."[2]

I thought of a story about a child who asked three experienced baseball umpires to explain how they distinguished a ball from a strike. The first umpire replied, "I call them as they are." The second replied, "I call them as I see them." The third replied, "They are as I see them." Psychotherapy is like that third umpire.

If Robert's present reality of staying stuck because of a gargantuan hearing-impairment cloud was "not that simple," my task was to show him other possibilities. I proposed to him that we needed to understand the complexity of influences that created "the cloud" in the first place and what kept it that way in the present. The last step would be to help him "reshape" that reality. He readily agreed.

Our next meeting occurred two weeks later. After Robert had responded to my typical opening question with "No, I don't have any specific place to begin," I opted to take the lead. "Let's figure out how you were taught to define your hearing loss as a massive cloud. For example, how did the kids who laughed at you back in elementary school help you define it?"

"As I told you, they laughed whenever I would answer a question wrong. They thought I was out to lunch all of the time, you know?"

"Did you believe them—that you were out to lunch?"

"Not at first. But after a while it sort of got to me and I began to believe them. I felt reduced to nothing. I guess I can remember many people—my mom, dad, teachers and friends—teaching me, as you say, that being hard of hearing meant being inferior. So I guess I was taught to feel stupid."

"It sounds like you were taught to view your hearing loss as a sort of package deal: that it comes with a massive cloud, with being out to lunch, not too bright, or reduced to nothing. You were taught to attach all that baggage to your disability. That's your internal, emotional handicap."

Robert nodded his head and exhaled a deep breath. I could tell he was consumed with sadness. We were silent for a moment.

"It must have been tough at school," I finally offered. "What did you do?"

"I tried to find the darkest corner of the room to hide. Sometimes literally, sometimes just by how I acted.

"And what did your classmates and teachers do when you hid?" I asked.

"Some laughed, and some poked fun at me. I guess they felt sorry for me. I knew I didn't get asked difficult questions. Maybe my teachers didn't want to embarrass me. But I knew what they were thinking—that I was some kind of defect."

"But that wasn't the case at all. Your intellect, personality, competence, etc. weren't defective—only your ears were. I'm very sorry that they chose to ignore you. They didn't have to ignore you—but they did."

Robert thought about that for a moment and then looked up at me, now making solid eye contact. I had said something that hit a nerve. Slowly, he nodded his head, and instead of criticizing his own behavior, he questioned the behavior of another. "You're right," he replied. "They didn't have to leave me hiding in the corner. They should have known what was going on!"

Now his voice contained a hint of anger, even of indignation. Rather than passively accept and internalize his teachers' neglect in a self-depreciatory manner—being out to lunch, stupid, reduced to nothing, etc.—he began to "give" some of the culpability back to them.

"Yes they definitely should have been more supportive," I quickly affirmed. "You were in a lot of pain and didn't have a way to share it so you hid. You were troubled but not troubling. So they didn't notice you. Everybody including your teachers didn't get the meaning of your behavior."

I imagined a common sequence: Robert felt inadequate in school and "hid in the corner"; his peers and teachers avoided him; he felt more inadequate and hid even more; others avoided him more. How that vicious cycle started is one of those "chicken or egg" questions: you continually act and react to your environment which, in turn, continually acts and reacts to you. It is like a dance. It requires at least two partners who coordinate each step. Stated differently, in a "dance," the culpability is shared: no one is solely to blame.

It was tempting to continue amplifying his teachers' part of that dance—what they could have and should have done—as it would provide Robert with an opportunity to explore his anger, but I was afraid that such "teacher bashing"—while the content may be valid—would have had the paradoxical effect of making his teachers and other authority figures seem more powerful, thereby reducing Robert to feeling even less empowered. Now it seemed more fruitful to help him explore his steps of the dance, both past and present.

He had already identified his own behavior of hiding in grade school which had made it easy for others to avoid and belittle him. But he could not change the past. So I asked him to explore his present-day behavior: "I understand more how, as a child, you hid in a corner and, in a sense, helped train people to define who you were. What do you do now?"

"I just feel really lost, under pressure, and, as I told you before, I'm petrified in groups."

"And what do you do now to show that?" I continued.

"I guess I withdraw. I sort of hide, like I did as a kid."

Robert made that important connection between his past and present. Since elementary school, his fear of looking stupid prevented him from asking for clarification of conversations that he did not understand. By Robert's own admission, he was the epitome of what has been called passing or the smile and nod syndrome—pretending to understand what others were saying. Both his past and present modus operandi were not to be in the world but to look at the world. Stated differently, he habitually looked at "Trivial Pursuit cards" rather than risk losing the game.

I simply piggy-backed on his astute observation and emphasized what he could change. "Like you, I'm struck by how similar your present dance is to your past dance, and by how you actually, in a sense, train people to look down on you. Your withdrawing and looking dumbfounded helps them think you are, in your words, out to lunch."

"Yeah, and after a while, I think that so many people can't be wrong."

"Exactly," I agreed. "Except that so many people in fact can be wrong. And believing their 'wrong' evaluations of you has devastating consequences for your self-esteem." Robert internalizing other peoples' negative evaluations of him had caused him to feel inferior and to act the part. Thoughts cause feelings which cause behavior. A basic tenet of cognitive therapy.[3, 4]

In this manner, Robert unwittingly encouraged people to reinforce the emergence of his internal handicap, his "unnecessary baggage."

"Can you change what you do when you don't understand something—your part of the so-called dance?" I asked. "You know, get rid of some bad, learned habits like when you smile and nod or look at Trivial Pursuit cards?"

"That's easy on paper," he instinctively replied. "But do you know how it feels to jump in a conversation and say something that has nothing to do with what people are talking about?"

"No, please tell me."

"It's humiliating!" he proclaimed. "I remember even watching my grandmother who became deaf. She always used to say things that were way off the subject. We all laughed at her! Boy, now I know how she must have felt!" Robert kept shaking his head.

"How must she have felt?" I asked.

"Humiliated, embarrassed, inept, stupid, foolish, scared." Robert had no shortage of words to describe this experience, whether about himself or projected on to his grandmother.

But unlike his grandmother, who unabashedly entered any conversation no matter what people might think of her, Robert evaluated a social gathering as a success if nobody asked "can you hear me?" and if everybody treated him exactly like everybody else. Convincing others that he was, in his words, "normal" took on greater importance than enjoying himself and learning from others. Whatever the cost, he needed to maintain his persona of having no disability. I am what I appear to others.

However, passing would not succeed for a variety of reasons. It required enormous amounts of energy which depleted his psychological resources. He complained of constant exhaustion and headaches. He would often inevitably respond incorrectly to what he thought someone said. Finally, his speech was different than that of hearing persons, prompting many people to comment on his foreign accent. For these reasons, he correctly perceived that other people saw through his "veneer" of acting like a hearing person. It felt to Robert like a certain death—the imminent outcome of his Trivial Pursuit nightmare.

The accumulated effects of attempting to "pass for a hearing person" inevitably caused Robert to suffer from not only self-depreciation, but also self hatred in the form of guilt and shame. At some level, he had to make sense out why he needed to pass. As he put it, "it almost seems that, after so many years of passing, I must have something awful to hide—like I'm a bad person."

I asked Robert to consider whether, at some level of awareness, he might be thinking the following algorithm to himself:

People who lie are bad.
I lie about understanding people.
Therefore I am bad.

Robert frantically nodded his head, obviously identifying with these statements. How ironic it was that Robert pretending that he had no disability worsened his internal handicap.

As our weekly sessions continued, he appeared to be enjoying our exploration. He often referred back to how his "lying about understanding people" caused him immense shame, "like I'm a really bad person." He recalled being punished as a child for telling lies. "The punishments weren't that bad," he recalled, "but what really hurt was feeling like a bad boy!"

I decided to take our discussion one step further by asking Robert to consider an elaborated corollary of that earlier algorithm. "After a period of time and several repetitions, your conclusion of 'therefore I'm bad' becomes sort of an independent entity—a self evident truth: 'I am bad because I am bad.' You then gather evidence, saying to yourself something like 'I'm bad because I did X, Y, Z.' Finally, as you grow up and your language becomes more advanced, you replace the 'I am bad' with more grown-up phrases, such as 'I am unsophisticated, dumb, ugly, inept.'

"At the same time, your negative thoughts about yourself get reinforced by others. As you know, many hearing people easily lose patience when asked to repeat themselves and to accommodate the special needs of another. Thus, you—like many people—may think that 'I am bad (or other negative attributes) because other people react to me as bad; therefore I must be bad.'"

"Okay, I'm done," I announced, as I sat back in my seat waiting for Robert's comments.

"Hey, doc," he smirked, "I haven't heard you talk that much since we met! You must have had a second cup of coffee this morning!"

We laughed. (I typically become "doc" after making what I have come to call "didactic outbursts.") "I guess I'm a frustrated teacher," I admitted. "Could you personalize my speech? Tell me what, if anything, felt relevant to you?"

Robert shifted positions slightly in his chair, as if to decide whether to say nothing, to tell me the short version of his reactions, or to tell me the whole story. He decided on the latter. "Because you gave me a speech, now it's my turn." He paused, took a deep breath and began, this time in a soft, somber voice: "To be perfectly honest with you, I often see myself as a little boy who hasn't grown up. I don't allow many people to see the real me, because, if they did, I fear they would somehow shit on me. Just the other day, I was at a party and someone told a joke. Not being able to pick up the innuendoes or the tone, all I heard were words, and I didn't catch the impact of the joke. But I decided to take a chance—just that once—and ask him 'Would you repeat that again?' (He was a good friend.) But he wouldn't repeat it. He said it wasn't important. What he meant was I wasn't important. And that's exactly how I feel."

From this experience and many others like it, Robert's disability of hearing loss "spread" to become internalized as a handicap of feeling "unimportant," like "other people are ten feet tall and I'm a little boy."

The term spread conjures up images for me of toxins being dumped into a body of water until it becomes totally polluted. Technically, spread refers to how much a disabled person views that disability as impeding not some aspects but all aspects of his/her functioning and being.[5] I recall a hard-of-hearing six-year-old girl who drew herself as one inch tall but with ears having a diameter of over one foot! If she were an adult, she would have verbally described this image as feeling totally consumed or "polluted" by her hearing loss. That is maximum spread.

Robert, too, appeared to feel totally "polluted" by his deafness. It was as if it rendered him a helpless, disempowered victim of circumstance—without any options. Like a massive hearing-impairment cloud.

It was time for us to more directly decrease the spread of his disability. Since he had begun to understand more how people in the past had taught him to feel handicapped, we could now more profitably modify his handicapping beliefs in the present. "Robert, you're absolutely right," I affirmed. "There's a lot about yourself and the world that you can't change. Some people undoubtedly do negate you, do shit on you. Oppression, discrimination, and racism, they're all alive and well in our world and they always will be. But your becoming empowered is not an all-or-nothing experience. Alongside what you can't change, you can change how you accept peoples' negation of you. You have control over that part."

Steven Covey, in his book *Seven Habits of Highly Effective People,* recommends a useful technique of listing what one can and cannot control.[6] It is essentially a version of the Serenity Prayer in 12-step programs. I suggested this task to Robert. It was no surprise to either of us that he began with the "cannot control" column, in fact, at lightening speed. His list threatened to fill up infinite reams of paper, obviously reflecting his pervasive sense of disempowerment and victimization.

The first four items of his Cannot Control list were

I can't appreciate classical music anymore
Discrimination
Being unable to join many conversations
Other people not caring.

It was interesting, but not at all uncommon, that the loss of music was at the top of his list. He later referred to classical music as having been "a soulful experience, as helping me along my spiritual path before becoming completely deaf." It had been his spirituality that had helped maintain his sense of basic integrity, far more than other psychological needs. He had practiced a type of Buddhist meditation to music. Consequently, it was that disruption of his spiritual needs that made his hearing loss so traumatic.

As Robert's list grew, I had the fantasy of it pressing down on his shoulders so much that he disappeared into the earth. When I asked him how he felt, he added his own metaphor of "feeling vaporized." We therefore both agreed that it was time to switch tasks. What could he control? Again, his response time was no surprise. Many moments slowly passed. He hesitated, fiddled with his pencil, and thought carefully before listing any items.

Finally, he listed

Using hearing aids
Educating people
Being assertive
Lobbying.

After scratching his forehead and fiddling with his pencil some more, he added several qualifications: "I can educate people but only those who wish to be educated." He noted the same for assertion, and the same for lobbying. "Many people don't give a shit," he lamented, "and that's something I can't control." Once again, his dark, enveloping cloud threatened to hide any glimpses of hope, but with some prompting, Robert began discussing how he nevertheless could choose friends who would validate his triumphs and pain. He added that those friends and interested others could also join hands and lobby against government officials who may indeed "not give a shit."

The process of "sifting out" control from noncontrol—regardless of what specific items come up—was the necessary medicine which helped Robert reduce the spread of his disability into an internal handicap. By expanding the list of what he could control, he was able to compartmentalize the overall effect of his hearing loss: "it does affect this, but it doesn't affect that." This process can also be described as "shifting gears," a descriptor that Social Worker Holly Elliott used with reference to her own hearing loss. In her words, "shifting gears is a process by which we choose change. Now that may seem crazy because we sure didn't 'choose' hearing loss. But we can choose how we manage it."[7]

As another example, consider the following letter from a woman who had become deaf as a young adult:

> If I identify too much with the impairment, it overtakes me—becomes a compulsion—when in itself it's neutral to my value as a person. So it is important for me to find value in myself elsewhere. Yet I do not want to deny I have or pretend about the impairment. It is a reality.

Robert was well on his way to finding value elsewhere. The next step was for him to perform some tasks on his own. First, I asked him to go swimming (which he loved), which necessitated taking off his hearing aids. I then instructed him not to avoid friends as he had done previously, but rather to actively seek them out and chat with them. It was a present-day opportunity of no longer "hiding in a corner," as he had done so many times in elementary school.

This kind of ritual is sometimes called "a corrective experience" or "*in vivo* desensitization." Robert and I preferred to call it "Facing Trivial Pursuit cards."

After some coaxing, he made a commitment to complete his therapy homework. "After all," he added, "what other people think doesn't have to be so important."

"Now you're talking! We can wish that others think highly of us, but we won't die if they don't. Approval from others does not always have to be a need."*

He nodded his head and smiled.

Two weeks later, he entered my office beaming with pride. He reported completing this task and was quite jubilant with his new found freedom. He exclaimed that "telling my friends that I couldn't hear them, that I wear hearing aids, and that I'm deaf was nowhere near as bad as my fantasy of how it would be!" Robert's realization reminded me of Franklin D. Roosevelt's observation, "the only thing we have to fear is fear itself."

At this time, Robert's initial success and enthusiasm compelled me to suggest a related, but more difficult task, namely, for him to purposely remove the batteries from his hearing aids before a relatively unimportant business meeting at work. I asked him to state to his colleagues that his batteries were dead and to be more assertive about getting clarification on what was being said.

Again, he returned the next week jubilant and with new insights. In particular, he was surprised at the respect he had received from his co-workers. "They made sure to include me. I was important enough."

As Robert continued to do what he had feared most, his world slowly but surely lost its vindictive power, or, stated more accurately, Robert had taken his power back! His abil-

---

*This is in contrast to children who need such approval, as they are largely molded by the environment around them.

ity to face and overcome his "worst fantasies" elevated his self-esteem. Whereas he previously was, in a sense, phobic about appearing to others as deaf, he again made the distinction between a disability and a handicap. In his words, "not hearing what someone says does not have to be a big deal." No longer ashamed, he emerged from his corner.

Another theme of our work had to do with helping Robert stop "waiting for Godot": for other people to initiate change. He realized that despite living in an oral/aural world that is often insensitive to his hearing loss, he, at least in part, was treated in a way that he taught others to treat him. He became more aware of the many choices he could actively make in his being in the world, even though he could neither change the whole world nor make his deafness go away. Now much more accepting of himself, he did not deem it as imperative that everybody respond affirmatively to him. He began to choose on whom to expend effort at achieving their acceptance and intimacy. He chose his small circle of friends.

Robert continued to experience increased vitality, now viewing each new challenge as an opportunity. He began new hobbies, such as oil painting and keeping a journal. He finally got the nerve to accept a lunch date with the woman at work whose advances had precipitated our first meeting a few months ago.

He also inquired about how to join S.H.H.H. (Self Help for the Hard of Hearing) and A.L.D.A. (Association of Late-Deafened Adults). Other ideas included perhaps lecturing in schools about common but unnecessary baggage with hearing loss. Maybe he would advocate for the rights of deaf people at his town hall, maybe even at the state level?

He was happy, in his words, "for the first time in years." We were both satisfied.

But one day Robert arrived at my office looking more distraught than I had seen him in a long time. His eyes were red and bloodshot, and his face was flushed. He had been crying for what he labeled as "crazy reasons." "Why just as everything in my life is going beautifully—I am happy, I've met wonderful people, I'm no longer in hiding—am I so sad?" he asked.

On the surface, his response to happiness seemed not crazy but at least unexpected or irrational. But his sadness represented a common and healthy therapeutic juncture that I had carelessly neglected to predict. Robert was beginning to grieve about how much happiness he had previously missed for so long, including how he had unwittingly participated in thwarting any progress toward that goal.

Although his constant "cloud" had previously caused him to feel depressed, it seldom caused him disappointment, acute pain, and torment; he could count on it. Not so now. The radiance of his emerging "sun" provided a stark contrast against the gloom of that "cloud." It was his newfound happiness that caused him to realize how depressed he had been and, in his words, "how many opportunities I had wasted." Fully experiencing new-found joy provided him for the first time with a yardstick with which to measure the emptiness that he had earlier denied.

He then let out his sadness that he had been embarrassed to show others. He sobbed. For what seemed like a long while, I sat with him, confident that words would follow. Between sobs, Robert shook his head and chanted over and over again, "what a waste, what a waste."

Although I was tempted to interject, "Yes, but now . . ." I restrained myself. Grieving his loss was an important part of his journey.

I remembered reading Plato's "Allegory of the Cave," a story about several men who had been tied up in a cave since birth with their backs toward a fire.[8] To them, ordinary reality consisted of only shadows. They accepted their reality without complaint until one man freed himself and saw the outside world for the first time. He then came back and reported to the men what they had been missing. As a result, they realized that their reality had indeed been constricted. Like Robert, they felt saddened by their loss of opportunities as well as joyous about their future.

Robert's grieving was his way of coming to terms with the unnecessary losses that he had sustained by remaining in his "cave" for so long. Robert said it best: "I am disabled, but I never had to be handicapped either by others or by myself."

——

After about four months, we agreed to stop meeting. He was feeling better, now accepting the duality of grieving his losses and relishing his future. Plato would have been proud.

Several months later, Robert requested another appointment. He brought in a large canvas covered with paper. Slowly and carefully, he unwrapped what he warned me was his first attempt at oil painting. His face beaming, he unveiled the culmination of how he had spent much of his free time. The painting brought tears to our eyes. It was a portrait of an angel.

He also had some important news about his recurring, Trivial Pursuit dream: "As before, I was leaving my house when suddenly the whole world became a Trivial Pursuit board. And everybody became Trivial Pursuit cards. But unlike before, when one of the cards tried to force me to answer the questions correctly, I stared at it and said 'I won't play your game anymore. But I'll teach you one of my own!'"

We both nodded our heads and smiled.

Notes

1. Ramsdell, D. A. (1978). The psychology of the hard-of-hearing and deafened adult. In H. Davis & S. R. Silverman, *Hearing and deafness* (4th edit.). New York: Holt, Rinehart & Winston.

2. Montalvo, B. (1976) Observation of two natural amnesias. *Family Process,* 15, 333–342.

3. Trychin, S. (1991). *Manual for mental health professionals: Part 2. Psycho-social challenges faced by hard-of-hearing people.* Washington, DC: Gallaudet University Press.

4. Meichenbaum, D. (1977). *Cognitive-behavior modification: An integrative approach.* New York: Plenum Publishing Corp.

5. Wright, B. A. (1960). *Physical disability: A psychosocial approach.* New York: Harper & Row.

6. Covey, S. (1989). *Seven habits of highly effective people.* New York: Simon & Schuster.

7. Elliott, H. (1986). Acquired hearing loss—shifting gears. *SHHH,* November/December, 23–25.

8. Grube, G. M. A. (Trans.) (1974). *Plato: The republic.* IN: Hockett Pub.

CHAPTER FIVE

Between Two Worlds

No matter what I did, Mary felt misunderstood. "How do you feel? Tell me more about that. It must be tough for you. Are you sad? Angry? Lonely?" To each of my queries, she would shake her head in mild disgust and complain that I wasn't taking her needs seriously enough. Mary was seventeen years old and a sophomore. She became hard-of-hearing shortly before puberty.

Her parents had ordered her to see a specialist in hearing loss, following one of a seemingly endless series of family fights about wearing her hearing aids. At that time, I directed an agency that served a Deaf clientele and I was heavily involved in learning American Sign Language and about Deaf culture. Although I do not have a hearing loss and had never before provided therapy for a hard-of-hearing person, I accepted the referral from Mary's mother who considered my qualifications as "close enough."

Mary was forthright about letting me know that therapy was not her idea. "This is stupid," was her frequent appraisal of the situation. She typically appeared depressed and complained about all the cliques at school, a mainstream setting in which there were "a few" Deaf students. Even though she was not involved in any extra curricular activities, because she stated she "needed as much time as possible to study," her grades were F's and D's. Her teachers admonished her for not working up to her potential and they wondered whether she had Attention Deficit Disorder.

"I'm not like deaf or hearing people. I don't fit in anywhere! You don't get it, do you?" she complained.

"Help me understand," I offered.

"I've tried but you ignore how I feel."

"So tell me more about not having friends."

"You don't get it, do you? You don't understand. Nobody understands me," she again complained.

"I get that you're unique, not like other people, that you're lonely, that you want more friends, that you fight with your parents. . . ."

"You don't get it!"

We were going around in circles. It was our sixth meeting.

I privately asked myself what adolescent, or adult for that matter, does not feel ignored or misunderstood? Mary had a lot going for her. She was bright, excelled in athletics, was well liked, and had good social skills. She appeared to be dealing with her hearing loss well. She had good speech, and good lip-reading skills. The receptionist referred to her as "that very nice young woman." I viewed my role as providing supportive therapy to help her get through what I judged to be a normal developmental stage of adolescence.

During this time period, my agency began advertising a conference that we emphasized was designed specifically for "Deaf and hard-of-hearing persons." Minutes before my next meeting with Mary, I received an inquiry from a prominent community leader who had just received our brochure. He asked "How is your conference specifically designed to include hard-of-hearing persons? What kind of assistive listening devices do you have?"

I was embarrassed to admit that all we had planned for was an American Sign Language interpreter. We had ignored the unique needs of the hard-of-hearing audience, who for the most part were not ASL users. Instead, we focused on the needs of the ASL-fluent, culturally Deaf audience. I thanked him for calling and said I'd get to work on it right away.

And now I was with Mary. Once again she, too, complained that I did not take her needs seriously.

But this time I finally got it.

I asked her to stand with both her arms outstretched and imagine that she was being pulled from both sides. As she swayed back and forth, I asked her to make one side the hearing world and the other side the Deaf world—and to continue being pulled in both directions. As she enacted this scenario, back and forth, back and forth, she grimaced. For the first time, she began to cry. We both stood there for an instant, almost in shock that this seemingly "simple" exercise could release so much pain.

The Pull Toward the Hearing World

From an audiologic perspective, the effects of a moderate hearing loss seem less problematic than the effects of a profound hearing loss. A person with a moderate or moderate-to-severe hearing loss, as measured in decibels across a certain frequency range, is typically said to be hard-of-hearing. An individual with a profound or severe-to-profound hearing loss is usually said to be deaf. This is implied by one definition of a hard-of-hearing person as "one who, generally with the use of a hearing aid or other assistive device, has residual hearing sufficient to enable *successful* (my emphasis) processing of linguistic information through audition."[1]

The pull toward the hearing world is a natural consequence of how well a hard-of-hearing person is able to function in situations among hearing persons. Or stated a bit more negatively, it is a consequence of how effectively one can exude a facade of being *un*impaired. Communication is often effective in one-to-one situations and in some small groups. Furthermore, many persons with a moderate hearing loss develop good oral skills, lip-reading skills, the use of residual hearing, and a command of English.

It is also common for such persons to identify with the basic values and interests of the hearing world. If their hearing loss was adventitious, i.e., acquired, they may have had normal or close-to-normal hearing for some part of their lives. Even if their hearing loss was congenital, they remain able to participate in many cherished auditory-based activities, for example, music or radio.

Mary often said "I feel like a hearing person. I belong in that world. Sure I have a hearing loss but, for the most part, I do just fine." She often appeared for our meetings wearing tee-shirts depicting various rock groups. She would regularly accuse me of being stuck in the past for attending Grateful Dead concerts.

In fact, her one solace was that she was not profoundly deaf. Each time she felt humiliated for any lip-reading faux pas, she felt relief that "at least I'm not that bad off." She had recurring fears of someday "selling sign language cards at Quincy Market Place," a tourist area in Boston. She did not view the Deaf community as a cultural minority, as "a difference to be accepted." Instead, she viewed deafness with a mixture of pity and contempt.

She sometimes performed for me her dramatic mockery of Deaf people using American Sign Language, describing it as a cross between Moe of the Three Stooges and "a mental retard." Rather than appreciating ASL as an intricate and beautiful language, she viewed it as inferior: "ASL is boring . . . I can't express my thoughts; after all, Deaf people, you know, use only one sign for the words 'wonderful,' 'fantastic,' 'magnificent,' 'extraordinary,' 'marvelous' . . . it's boring." Although I knew the reverse situation also occurs when there are many ASL signs for an English word, I was not surprised Mary had this misperception.

Barriers to the Hearing World

Deafness has been called the most invisible disability, but perhaps this dubious distinction should be shared. The several profound ramifications of being hard-of-hearing seem "more invisible" in some ways, as they are often unrecognized by the lay public. Invisible or not, the effects of moderate hearing loss all too frequently render one's experience in the hearing world as tenuous and as fraught with barriers as profound deafness.

Communication frustration in some ways seems greater for hard-of-hearing people than congenitally deaf people. The latter, having experienced since birth the insurmountable task of fully and easily understanding spoken English, are often more resigned to this limitation. Furthermore, if the sound is emanating out of eyesight, they often are unaware of its occurrence. In contrast, hard-of-hearing people are more aware that they are missing something. Hard-of-hearing people often exert a tremendous amount of effort trying to understand what others are saying, but find themselves feeling lost and resorting to guesswork. There are endless examples: oral group conversations, cash registers without a clear visual read-out, telephone operators, and, beginning in adolescence, group gatherings in dimly lit rooms.

Mary, for example, reported that "I often almost understand what people are saying, but not quite." The harder she tried, the harder it would become. In her words, "I can't even begin to explain how scared and nervous I get; it's beyond words." Psychologist Edna Levine provides these words:

> Countless young hard-of-hearing people live in daily terror of being caught in the joshing camaraderie of a hearing group; of being singled out in games; of being called on in class; and, worst of all,

missing the 'sweet nothings' whispered into their ears on dates.[2]

Frustration and anxiety often lead to withdrawal. As one hard-of-hearing adolescent eloquently put it, "I can tell the difference between AC/DC and The Police, but understanding what my friends are saying is a pain in the ass. So I just hang out, you know, not talking to people but just looking cool."

In the words of a hard-of-hearing, middle-aged man

Even today, I have to fight, to battle, with myself to go to a party, to any kind of gathering. I still haven't overcome that. Sometimes friends will say they're going to have a cook out or a party and ask if I would like to come. I'd say "sure, fine, no problem." But as the days and hours draw closer, I tend to get a little bit negative, to the point that I would become almost depressed by the fact that I had to go to this thing. Who wants to go to such a time-wasting thing anyway? You know, I just sort of create a black picture out there.

Although Mary thrived on parties, she also created a "black picture out there" and lived in daily terror. Even her solace of "at least I'm not deaf" brought no relief. Instead, it fueled her fears of losing more hearing. In contrast to profoundly deaf people who, for the most part, know that their hearing loss is permanent, some hard-of-hearing people, like Mary, experience frequent fluctuations in their level of hearing. Consequently, audiologic visits precipitated dread and fear for Mary. In addition, a common head cold or earache, which naturally attenuates one's hearing, was also frightening for her. In Mary's words, "there is always a threat that I'll be expelled from the hearing world and sentenced to be in the Deaf community."

Hard-of-hearing persons can almost "become" hearing but not quite. For this reason, as Mary stood with her arms outstretched, she swayed away from the hearing world and toward the Deaf world.

The Pull Toward the Deaf World

"After all," Mary reasoned, "deaf people also have an auditory disability." From an audiologic perspective, she was quite correct. Both deaf and hard-of-hearing persons may wear hearing aids and attend speech therapy, they may demand "reasonable accommodations" at work or school, and they are often labeled by hearing people as "hearing impaired." Both groups certainly know what it is like to be "outsiders in a hearing world."[3]

Mary also emphasized that "deaf people also understand what prejudice is like because they, too, have experienced more than their fair share of oppression." She recalled countless examples of hearing people dismissing her with "Never mind, what we were talking about wasn't important; just try harder to lip-read." Common stories.

In fact, both groups are frequently subject to overt and subtle job discrimination and often have to fight relentlessly for many basic human rights, even after the passage of the Rehabilitation Act and the Americans with Disabilities Act. For this reason, Deaf and hard-of-hearing people often join hands politically to lobby in the larger, hearing world. Massachusetts, for example, has the Massachusetts Commission for the *Deaf and Hard-of-Hearing* (italics added) which received its initial funding through the joint efforts of both communities.

There were perhaps other reasons why Mary swayed toward the Deaf world. Some hard-of-hearing people are attracted to the Deaf community, not out of a sense of comaraderie, but out of a need to "help." They incorrectly view the Deaf community as ill-equipped and of lesser stock than hard-of-hearing people. They believe that the Deaf need their help to function well in the hearing world.

In contrast, other hard-of-hearing people may idealize Deaf people and therefore wish to identify with them in some way. On television and in the movies, Deaf people are sometimes portrayed as idealized giants whose skills and prowess are impossible for the average Deaf person to achieve. Marlee Matlin, a recent and popular example, is seen on prime-time television as a "Deaf" person who not only understands lip-reading at fifty paces, but also understands someone signing to her back.[4]

Some hard-of-hearing people become intrigued with American Sign Language. This may be the result of taking a course in "Sign," from having attended a signed play, or from having met Deaf people in a bar, Deaf club, or other social gathering. Unlike Mary who had scorned ASL as "a boring language," many hard-of-hearing people are captivated by it. One hard-of-hearing man, for example, worked with Deaf people as a result of his interest in ASL.

There are many other pulls toward the Deaf world, but after learning their language and attending Deaf events, some people nevertheless remain outsiders. Others go the next step and choose to become members of the Deaf community by also adopting the attitudes, norms and values of Deaf culture. They happily learn that one's acceptance into the Deaf community depends on several factors, including one's self-proclaimed Deaf identity and fluency with American Sign Language.[5] Whether one has a profound hearing loss is relatively unimportant.

Barriers to the Deaf World

I am struck, however, by how often the theme of feeling peripheral to the Deaf community emerges from the sentiments of hard-of-hearing people. They seem acutely aware of the distinction between being accepted by the Deaf community as a Deaf person (spelled with a capital "D" to indicate membership in the Deaf culture/community) and being labeled as a deaf person (spelled with a small "d" to indicate that one has a hearing loss but is not a member of the Deaf culture/community).[6]

The reasons for these peripheral feelings are complex. The cohesiveness of the Deaf community may be one factor. As with any oppressed minority group with a history of defamation and discrimination, culturally Deaf people may be somewhat guarded with outsiders and more cohesive within their community. A hard-of-hearing adult expressed a common sentiment: "I envy the Deaf community's togetherness, their support of each other, Deaf cultural events, The National Theater of the Deaf, The National Association of the Deaf, their sense of identity. But I don't sign, never have learned, and I'm not Deaf. So I'm not one of them."

As another hard-of-hearing man put it

> I don't really feel like I belong with Deaf community people. I sense they have a great need, great enthusiasm, but I don't really understand them. I don't know how to relate to them other than to try to be warm, but that's as far as I can go with them. Although we're both labeled as "hearing impaired"—and, by the way, I feel that's a terrible term (it should never be used, really)—the hard-of-hearing are in the normal hearing world. The Deaf go to the Deaf culture, which is increasingly becoming sophisticated, and find ways to cope with their particular problems. I don't use their sign language. It's two different worlds entirely. Culturally and every other way!

Many hard-of-hearing people attempt to learn ASL, but report feeling overwhelmed and frustrated. Others actually fear sign language. As one woman said, "I know it's silly but I find myself thinking that if I learn ASL, I'll lose more of my hearing and become deaf." This is an example of magical thinking. Most of us engage in some form of it, illogical as it may be. As an example, when there are airplane turbulence, I always look at the seat in front of me to stabilize the plane. This strategy works every time!

For whatever reason, many people give up learning ASL. Some compensate for their frustration or fear by scorning it. Recall Mary's dramatic mockery of sign language. Still others do not learn ASL from a Deaf teacher (who is typically far more proficient than a hearing teacher), but learn an English-based visual-coding system which is part of the hearing, not Deaf, culture.

In Mary's case, she swayed toward the Deaf world only to a certain point. Then she retreated: "my basic values and interests are with hearing people; I just don't feel Deaf." Now as she stood with her arms outstretched, she swayed away from the Deaf world and toward the hearing world.

Between Two Worlds

Mary continued to sway back and forth between two worlds, now with tears streaming down her face. Then she abruptly stopped, gazed toward the ceiling, clasped her hands together, and ever so tentatively made eye contact with me. In a soft, almost confessional-like manner she murmured "I don't fit in either world."

She eventually sat down, took a deep breath, and looked at me, seemingly hoping that I finally understood her longstanding struggle. Perhaps to ensure that I got it, she made a further comment: "I feel ignored. Hearing people view me as too deaf. Deaf people view me as too hearing. I wish I was one or the other."

But there was no need for further clarification. By that time, I got it. Mary had been consumed by a private tug-of-war that nobody, including me, had noticed or understood. I felt a deep sense of compassion for her and gratitude that she had taken the risk of revealing her inner torment to me. Our dialogue could now be at a deeper, more intimate level.

What are the effects of one's family and social and professional networks ignoring this internal tug of war? Consider the following letter which was sent to me from a woman, age twenty-five:

> I have a severe bilateral sensorineural hearing loss and wear binaural hearing aids. I feel this "tug of war" both at work and in my personal life. I often feel like saying, "to hell with the hearing world, I'll just be deaf (with a small d)." Since I am unfamiliar with Deaf culture and the Deaf community, I would not belong. This, coupled with my fear of isolation from the "hearing world" has kept me struggling to remain in the hearing community.
>
> The resulting feeling of being ignored often mounts so substantially that anger takes over. I find myself blaming my normal hearing friends for not helping me to participate more effectively. 'Why can't they sense my frustration and come to my rescue?' I often ask myself. It is getting difficult for me to maintain a healthy attitude and to hang on to my self confidence in these instances. How can I make significant others understand my struggle?
>
> My tolerance for having to sit back and observe rather than participate in group conversations continues to lessen. I feel I am beginning to withdraw from social situations to spare me the inevitable frustration that develops. This scares me tremendously.

Mary also vacillated between feeling angry and scared. Her "sort-of boyfriend" had just asked her to the high school prom, an event that her older sister had assured her "would make you a woman." (Mary's sister had lost her virginity at the after-prom party, a secret that she had shared only with Mary.)

"Most people would be thrilled!" Mary lamented. Although "Eddie" was usually "more sensitive than most of them," his advice to her about how to have a good time at that dark, noisy, impossible-for-lip-reading event was to "just deal with it."

"He doesn't get it, does he?" I offered.

"He sure doesn't! It's a snobbish, stuck-up thing to say! He should stick it . . ." she proclaimed in anger. She now viewed me as on her side.

But then she thought for a moment and spoke from the opposite side of her ambivalence: "But he's so cute. Many other girls are dying to go out with him. What if he tells me something at the prom I can't hear? I'll be laughed at. What if I can't follow what people say? What if my hearing aids squeal?" Right before my eyes, her anger became transformed into fear, mostly having to do with disappointing Eddie, whom she had previously deemed as stuck up. She became consumed by all the "what ifs." Her body began to shake.

Adolescent identity crisis. Without a stable sense of self — an emotional anchor—that one achieves in later adulthood, Mary continually vacillated between experiencing anger and experiencing fear, entitlement verses self-depreciation, and assertiveness verses passivity. One minute she would deem herself as popular, but then complain that "I have no friends." She would feel beautiful, but the next minute be "full of pimples." One day the world was awesome, and the next day it was coming to an end because Eddie did not call. As her mother once complained, "I never know who's gonna wake up from her bed in the morning." The truth was, neither did Mary.

I was reminded of a research study of so-called "normal" adolescents.[7] They were asked to document their thoughts, feelings, and behaviors at random intervals for two weeks.

Thousands of protocols were then tabulated and summarized, and several typical "cases" were presented to a group of experienced clinicians for discussion. However, they were erroneously told that the subjects were adults, not adolescents. Almost all the clinicians rendered diagnoses of manic depression! What is normal for adolescents may be manic depression for adults!

In Mary's case, her mood fluctuations were attributable not to a psychiatric disorder but to a challenging mixture of hard-of-hearing and adolescent "Who am I? Where do I belong?" confusions. The dating issue was one of many examples. Her "sort-of" boyfriend was hearing. But another boy whom Mary categorized as "almost deaf" (he was audiologically hard-of-hearing) was very good looking, and "even better, he had his driver's license. . . ." Maybe she would go out with him? She secretly felt left out of "fun" Deaf community events, and only marginally engaged in activities with hearing groups.

Now that I finally understood her identity struggles, she was much more engaged in our work. Mary more openly discussed her social anxiety and sense of alienation from her peers, despite the fact that she was frequently invited to parties and sports events. No matter how busy she was, something was missing.

One day she reported a dream: "the door into the Deaf world was slammed shut and the door to the hearing world was left open only wide enough for me to peek in." Its meaning was clear. In Mary's words, "I feel lost, confused, lonely, in a void, in limbo."

Social worker Holly Elliott, who is deafened herself, described her version of feeling in limbo:

> Hearing people often think I am hearing because my speech is good; deaf people often think I am hearing because my signs are bad . . . we are caught between

incomprehensible speech on the one hand and in-comprehensible signs on the other. If only those hearies would talk more clearly! If only those deafies would sign more slowly! Who's taking care of us?[8]

In Mary's case, her parents were trying their best to take care of her. But Mary elected to hide her anxieties and vulnerabilities from them. Instead, she showed them only her outward irritability and obstinacy. As I now had a more complete understanding of Mary's inner world, I began to become much more curious about what was behind the almost never-ending family conflicts.

Although I was primarily providing individual therapy to Mary, we had taken care to schedule intermittent meetings with her parents so I could get a more complete understanding of family issues and hopefully diffuse some conflicts. It was vital to avoid a common pitfall of colluding with Mary against her parents.

One day her mother called to schedule one of their fights in my office (I imagined it as "round #239"), this time about making a routine audiologic appointment. Mary had requested that her parents come to our session. Her reason was predictable and finally volunteered to me during an individual visit after much prodding: "I want you to convince them to get off my back."

It was a set up if I ever saw one! I suggested a more reasonable goal: "How about meeting with you and them to figure out different ways of fighting?"

"Fair enough," she sighed.

Two weeks later, I invited Mary and her parents in from the waiting room. To my surprise, "round #239" had already ended by the time of our meeting. They had just visited the audiologist. No change in Mary's hearing status. But now they were arguing about school placement.

Her father's position was clear: "Mary's too smart for

deaf people. She's now in a good mainstream school. She's in small classrooms with acoustic tiles and rugs, uses a phonic ear system, and has excellent teachers who also know about hearing impairment. She should stay there and become more confident about using support services. We'll even get her an oral or sign language interpreter if she wants one. It's a hearing world out there, you know. It's tough! She's gotta learn to assert herself and. . . ."

"But she's not hearing and she's always at a disadvantage with hearing peers," pleaded her mother. She then presented her position: "A school for the Deaf or program with other hard-of-hearing kids would give her a peer group of kids like her. And she could learn signing as a second language because some of her teachers would sign. And the whole school would already know about hearing impairment. Mary wouldn't have to be the guinea pig anymore!"

"Maybe not, but Mary should be in a normal public school," retorted her father. "Even some of the deaf programs said so." He was referring to some of the bicultural, bilingual, Deaf programs who had said that Mary would not fit in because she was "too hearing."

Mary's mother had a predictable comeback: "But public school teachers aren't always going to be sensitive to her needs! Even the principal thinks that she'll do just fine by having only a few support services. He thinks she's a hearing person, but she isn't!"

"Don't forget," her dad began, "about all the residual hearing she has and—"

"You're forgetting Mary's hearing loss," her mom interrupted.

At that instant, Mary and I smiled at each other. It was a deja vu to several weeks ago when she had first stood up, outstretched her arms, and enacted her internal tug of war experience. Her own ambivalence about affiliating with the

Deaf and hearing worlds was now being enacted in front of her.

The "Between Two Worlds" struggle is frequently enacted between parents of hard-of-hearing students. In the words of another mother:

> Many other parents like me find ourselves shunned by mainstream, hearing programs because our children aren't "deaf." The schools don't recognize that we also have concerns regarding the cost of hearing aids, speech therapy, etc. and that our children require lots of support services which set them apart from "normal children." Our kids, likewise, don't fit in schools for "deaf children" because they're not deaf, they're hard-of-hearing. Somewhere in between both extremes.

Mary's mother focused more on the Deaf extreme, her father more on the hearing extreme. (Recall that it was her mother who had originally made the referral to me, stating that my deafness qualifications were adequate.) Her mother was half-right. Knowledge of deafness is a necessary qualification for treating hard-of-hearing clients. But in support of her father, it is also important to be aware that many hard-of-hearing people are affiliated more toward the hearing than toward the Deaf world.

Her parents continued to debate each other. As it escalated and became more heated and fast-paced, it struck me that Mary was more an observer than a participant. She got a neck ache trying to lip-read the ping-ponging back and forth. Undoubtedly, she missed much of it.

That pattern was important to change. I smiled at Mary and asked "So, by the way—since this is about you—what do you think?"

She shifted uncomfortably in her chair, obviously having been at least partially content to be only a spectator of the

"Deaf–hearing debate" between her parents. I wondered aloud whether one reason for her internal experience of feeling "in limbo" between these two worlds reflected not only her cultural identity confusion, but also her fear of betraying either one of her parents. It seemed like a catch 22.

In answer to that question, Mary shook her head, but not convincingly. It was clear that she did not want to openly state her position.

I wondered how entrenched her parents were in their opposing views. Therefore, I asked both of them to rate their degree of certainty of their respective positions on a one to ten scale, with ten as "most sure." Judging from the persuasiveness of their "opening and closing arguments" (which rivaled those of the best of attorneys), I privately predicted ratings of either a nine or a ten.

However, much to my surprise, and without much hesitation, Mary's mother volunteered a middle of the road rating of only six! And her father, after mulling it over a bit (I imagined in order to build up the suspense), gave a rating of only seven! Like Mary, they were also ambivalent!

Although it had at first seemed like a catch 22 situation—in which Mary thought that agreeing with one parent would be viewed by the other as collusion—in fact all three of them were privately ambivalent!

Now I asked each of them to continue their debate but to reverse positions. (I remember this from high school as a typical debate-coaching strategy.) After some initial laughter and awkwardness, each began to argue their new positions as persuasively as before!

After several minutes elapsed, I finally said, "You know, Mary, you don't have to worry about betraying either your mom or your dad. It looks like they'll partially agree with you either way."

She nodded her head and smiled. I imagined a heavy weight lifted from her shoulders.

Our next individual meeting occurred two weeks later. The frequency of family fighting had lessened somewhat. In particular, Mary commented that "my parents don't seem to fight about deaf versus hearing stuff so much anymore." However, she reported one "huge battle" over the use of the car during a recent snow storm. After we both acknowledged sarcastically how "tough and utterly unreasonable it was that she didn't get the family car during a huge blizzard and ice storm," we moved on to discuss other "relevant matters."

With her face beaming, Mary announced that she had to make "a big decision." It seemed that she had been asked to the prom by another boy in addition to Eddie—the one who she had previously labeled as "almost deaf."

"Remember I told you about Andy before—the one who has his own car? He's real cute! I don't know whether to go to the prom with him or with Eddie." She then added, in what looked like a staged matter-of-fact manner, that "Andy also said he'd teach me some secret signs."

"Making a decision is much different than being a victim of your previous tug-of-war experience. What changed?" I asked.

It felt significant to me that much of Mary's experience of herself in the world up to now had been in a passive, "limbo" position between the Deaf and hearing groups and between her mother and father. Now that her parents openly supported her no matter what group she joined, she appeared to become unstuck.

"I dunno what changed," she responded. "It just feels different. Not everything has a reason you know!" she reminded me. "But I can tell you—if you really *have to* analyze everything to death" she smiled, "that I need friends who really understand me!"

I smiled and nodded my head, thinking of her urgent requests to be understood during our initial meetings.

Beyond the Tug-of-War:
In Search of a Reference Group

Although Mary had exuded a persona of being autonomous, self-determined, and independent, she, like the rest of us, had a strong psychological need for peers and role models who "are like me." For the first time, she openly admitted her needs to feel that essential alikeness with a hard-of-hearing peer community. For now, that peer would be Andy. It seemed that they were "almost going out with each other!"

One day, Mary and her parents were invited to meetings sponsored by Self Help for the Hard of Hearing (S.H.H.H.) and Association of Late-Deafened Adults (A.L.D.A.). Mary put up her characteristic modicum of resistance as she predicted it was for "boring adults." But, her parents invited Andy along, too, promising him and Mary the use of the family convertible the following night. They readily agreed to those terms.

Although, in each of these groups, all the members were adults—often many years older than Mary—she nevertheless experienced a strong sense of identification, of that "essential alikeness." Many of the deafened and hard-of-hearing adults she met had experienced their hearing losses as teenagers, and they knew intimately the internal tug of war loneliness that Mary thought only she—and perhaps now Andy—had experienced.

Mary was also struck by how the hard-of-hearing people in these groups had taken the next step. By coming together and validating each other's experience, they had forged a solid "place" for themselves rather than existing in a void between two other "places." As the preamble to the Self Help for the Hard of Hearing constitution reads

> We are people who do not hear well, but are not deaf. We tend, increasingly, to be isolated. The existing pattern of community life lacks both means of

communication and institutions for us to solve our special problems and live normal lives. For too long, too
many of us have accepted a loneliness we are unable to
explain to our friends or even to our families. . . .[9]

Mary was no longer resigned to being stuck between the
Deaf and hearing worlds like she had been stuck between
her parents. She began to hang out with Andy a lot more
and now even attended deaf and hard-of-hearing social
gatherings. She learned enough signs so that they could
hold private conversations right in front of Mary's parents!

She also hung out with Eddie. "I'm not into going steady,"
she emphasized. Moreover, as Mary was becoming more comfortable with her alliances and identity, she also taught Eddie
some signs. She observed "I think he's finally getting it!"

Mary continued to transcend the tug of war. She had
found her world in which there were empathic others: people
who would validate her needs as a hard-of-hearing person, a
world that she could enter and leave as she pleased. Although
she continued to attend dark, noisy and impossible-for-lip-
reading school dances and outings, she no longer felt like a
"freak without a home." She did not have to be lonely any
more.

Her parents were initially thrilled. With progress, however, came new challenges. Now they fought about the use
of the TTY.* She would be on it "for hours!"

———

During one of our last visits, I recall commenting to Mary
that it was a shame she had not found a hard-of-hearing
peer group many years earlier.

I don't think so," she responded in a very adult, mature
manner. "For some people I've met who've lost their hearing, it's good for them to meet people like them—the

———

*Used by Deaf people, TTY is the acronym for teletypewriter, a commu-
nication device that uses phone lines.

sooner the better. But for me, I wasn't emotionally ready. I had to figure some stuff out first."

Her professorial tone made me smile, as I thought of how much she had taught me about the unique issues that hard-of-hearing people experience. Now she reminded me that timing is everything.

After about six months, it was time to say goodbye. We agreed to meet again at some point to either check in or do what is called in the profession "another piece of work." It would have been easier for me to end treatment only when Mary's life was stable, but that option reflected my own difficulty in letting go. Knowing that Mary was continuing her adolescence and entering adulthood meant facing many more crises and challenges.

Perhaps sensing my anxiety, she reminded me of another lesson about termination: "Mike, don't worry, I'll be okay!"

I said that I very much knew she would be okay and acknowledged my own difficulty in letting go. I admitted that it was tough to say goodbye to a cherished mentor.

Notes

1. Moores, D. F. (1982). *Educating the deaf: Psychology, principles and practices* (2nd ed.). Boston, MA: Houghton Mifflin Co.

2. Levine, E. S. (1981). *The ecology of early deafness: Guides to fashioning environments and psychological assessments.* New York: Columbia University Press.

3. Higgins, P. C. (1980). *Outsiders in a hearing world: A sociology of deafness.* Beverly Hills: Sage.

4. Hoffmeister, R. J., & Harvey, M. A. (1997). Is there a psychology of the hearing? In N. Glickman & M. A. Harvey (Eds.), *Culturally affirmative psychotherapy with deaf people.* New Jersey: Lawrence Erlbaum Associates.

5. Lane, H., Hoffmeister, R., & Bahan, B. (1996). *A journey into the deaf-world.* San Diego, CA: DawnSignPress.

6. Padden, C. (1980). The deaf community and the culture of deaf people. In *Sign language and the deaf community.* Silver Spring, MD: National Association of the Deaf.

7. Csikszentmhialyi, M., & Reed, L. (1984). *Being adolescent.* New York: Basic Books.

8. Luey, H.S. (1980). Between worlds: The problems of deafened adults. *Social work in Health Care.* 5 (3), 253–262.

9. Stone, H. W. (1985). Developing SHHH, a self-help organization. In H. Orlans (Ed.), *Adjustment to adult hearing loss.* San Diego, CA: College-Hill Press.

CHAPTER SIX

Presbycusis, Mortality, and Brussels Sprouts

Old people scare me. Norma, of course, didn't know that when I met her in the waiting room. She returned my handshake and very politely said "it's nice to meet you too." When I beckoned her into my office, she slowly and tentatively propelled herself up from her chair to a stooped, upright position.

She had not come willingly. Her two adult children—Marty, age fifty-four, and Joan, age fifty-two—also stood up on either side of her. They had made the appointment and had escorted her to our meeting. I imagined them dragging her, kicking and screaming, and now standing guard over their prisoner. After entering my office and making sure that Norma sat down in the chair furthest from the door, they took two seats that blocked the exit.

Norma had just celebrated her eightieth birthday.

Her children and several relatives threw a big bash at a local hotel. Over 100 people showed up, but Norma could not participate in most of the festivities due to presbycusis, a bilateral, high-frequency hearing loss that is typically age-related. She could not hear her children's toast, nor her grandchildren singing Happy Birthday.

"If only you would have worn your hearing aids," pleaded Marty and Joan in unison.

"Oh come now, it was a very nice party. It was very thoughtful of you," Norma retorted.

"Why won't you wear them?"

"Please don't worry about me. I'll be fine."

"You have to wear them! We bought them! We paid for them! They will help you hear! Why won't you wear them? Why? Why?"

The session had begun. They had battled for over two years, ever since Marty and Joan dragged her to an audiologist, who prescribed two binaural hearing aids. Top of the line. Sometimes Norma outright refused to wear her aids; other times she "misplaced them" or complained that they "didn't work properly." More pleading by her children lead to more passive or active refusal by Norma, which lead to more pleading. It was a cycle that had gone nowhere except to create mutual hostility and frustration.

It is scary to imagine the helplessness that comes with the so-called "golden years": sensory losses, health deterioration, loss of friends, and eventually loss of one's life. As much as Norma may not have been ready to see me as a psychologist, I was not emotionally ready to see her as a client. That occasion was a little over fifteen years ago when I had just begun my clinical practice. I had avoided taking any seminars on geriatrics with the rationalization that I could do that anytime when I got "older."

It seemed to me a cruel coincidence that I turned thirty years old only days after meeting Norma. Back then, thirty seemed old, and I recall feeling disgruntled because some of my colleagues, who were over forty or fifty years old, did not adequately sympathize. (At this writing, I am forty-five and realize how silly my complaints must have sounded.) However, it was at age thirty when it first dawned on me—on a visceral level—that my own life was finite. That crisis was enough. I was not ready to see myself fifty years down the road like her. Woody Allen said it best. When he was asked about the spiritual benefits of accepting his own mortality, he replied, "I have nothing against death, I just don't want to be there when it happens."

Norma portrayed an odd mixture of frailty and tenacity. She sat hunched over in her chair, seemingly burdened by her own weight and by her children's concerns. I noticed that she had slight hand tremors and imagined that they may have been due to medications, a neurological disorder, or anxiety. She clearly looked out of place in my office. In the middle of our meeting, as her children were reciting the history, she complained about missing "Wheel of Fortune."

That was Marty and Joan's cue to exclaim in unison, "But you can't even hear that program! Why don't you let us help you? Why don't you follow your audiologist's recommendations? Why don't you. . . ."

Round number two. This time she answered their "whys" with silence. She undoubtedly knew she could not hear well and that she could not do a host of other activities, but she could still piss off her children! Despite understanding their good intentions—and despite my own naiveté that hearing aids can help everyone with a hearing loss—I admired Norma's fortitude.

I thought of other stories illustrating fortitude in the face of helplessness. Victor Frankl wrote about prisoners of concentration camps who made rhythmic movements of their index fingers inside their pockets; it was the one thing the Nazis could not control. Many Deaf adults who had felt "imprisoned" in oral schools, where they had been punished for using American Sign Language, recall cherishing their sleep for similar reasons; "at least my dreams were my own."

The person in front of me in my office, however, was neither the victim of Holocaust torture nor oral school parochialism. I was observing two well-meaning children attempting to convince their mother to follow the cogent advice of a well-meaning audiologist. What's so bad about that? Why couldn't she just give hearing aids a chance?

I found myself formulating strategies with Joan and Marty—privately called "Operation Convince Norma to Wear Her Hearing Aids."

Family therapy became the battle arena. In preparation, I read about older people. At that time, the ageism in our culture infiltrated the field of geriatrics; for example, the popular assumption, typically of younger people, was that old people naturally fear death. In fact, recent research suggests that old people who achieve a certain level of what is called "psychological integrity," may not fear death per se.[1] Instead, their fear is that they will not have control over the timing and quality of their death: whether it will be sudden or lingering, painful or comfortable.[2]

I also learned about "interiority," defined as the inability to understand complex information and the unwillingness to deal with complicated and challenging situations. This was certainly Norma! At that time, I interpreted her refusal to wear hearing aids as her way of withdrawing from the environment she obviously found overwhelming or too complicated. It also seemed obvious to me at the time that her becoming less interior, i.e., being able to hear better, would necessitate her coming to terms with her own eventual death. I would come to correct that assumption later.

Upon researching strategies of increasing patient compliance, I found that physicians shared a common frustration: the typical patient compliance rate was only fifty percent and often much lower. Essentially, most doctors could predict whether their patients would comply with medical treatment by flipping a coin. Much of the literature explained that noncompliance—or nonadherence, as it is often called today—occurs because of a defective character of the individual, referred to as the "noncompliant personality."

Was this Norma? By her own admission, she was inflexible about appointment times (she insisted our meetings take place only between 2:00 and 4:00 pm for reasons unknown) and always sat in the same chair with the same stiff, rigid position, but she was not always that way. When I asked her about her earlier life (and to myself I added the phrase "before getting old"), she recounted numerous times of gaiety and spontaneity. She and both children agreed that, if anything, she had been a follower and gave in too much.

However, just as her personality had clearly changed, so had the context of her relationships. For most people, deteriorating health typically comes with a swarm of health-care professionals, each equipped with an arsenal of well-meaning advice and admonishments that "if you don't do so and so, you'll be sorry," and back up by persistent reinforcement of family members and friends. Pitted against this surge of help is a resistant patient, labeled as noncompliant, perhaps even mentally incompetent. Blame the victim.

Through my preparations for "Operation Convince Norma to Wear Her Hearing Aids," it became clear that people like Norma, who have a hearing loss as a result of presbycusis, may not follow audiologic recommendations for multifaceted and overlapping reasons. What follows are the results of my research:

1. **Hearing Aid Factors**

   Initial physical discomfort. Often referred to as the psycho-acoustic trauma.

   Prohibitive cost. Often this expense is not covered by insurance.

2. **Individual Psychological Factors**

   Denial of hearing loss. "The world is mumbling; it's not me."

   Level of comfort with dependency. How much one

is willing/able to tolerate needing an assistive device.

Level of comfort with stigma. The degree of concern about others thinking negatively about hearing aids.

Confusion about audiologic recommendations. Short-term memory capacity declines with age and in situations of increased anxiety, such as audiologic/doctor's appointments. This makes it more difficult to remember and/or follow complex audiologic directions.

Fine motor difficulties. Perceptual-motor and fine motor skills also decline with age. Therefore, older people may have difficulty manipulating the tiny controls on the hearing aid.

Hiding behind an acoustic barrier to the world. Older people often experience fatigue and depression because of a higher prevalence of neurologic disorders and medication side effects. Both cause a withdrawal from the world. Using hearing aids effectively strips this defense.

Mitigating feelings of powerlessness. Common methods include missing appointments; losing hearing aids—the "it flushed down the toilet phenomenon"; pitting conflicting recommendations of one audiologist against the other; and/or actively refusing treatment.

3. **The Relationship Between Audiologist and Client**

Distrust toward audiologist. For example, "I don't know what it is about him but . . ." or "All the audiologists I have met. . . ." Various symptoms or pathologies, such as tinnitus and vestibular disorders, may lead to heightened feelings of helplessness and therefore to increased suspiciousness or distrust.

Disagreement about appropriate treatment. Many consumers rely on other nonaudiologic treatments, i.e., acupuncture, herbal remedies, Christian Science, etc.

The necessary information was not provided. Too much jargon. In addition, the necessary information may not have been written down.

4. **The Relationships among Audiologist, the Consumer, and the Family**

Closed, rigid boundaries surrounding the consumer and family. An unspoken agreement within the family system to prohibit entry of others, including audiologists.

Power struggles between family members, audiologist, and the consumer. This is exemplified by Norma and her children. The consumer views first family members and then an audiologist as ganging up on him/her. The consumer therefore resists more.

Failure of an audiologist to ally with relevant family members. On the other hand, a consumer may rely on a particular family member's judgement, i.e., concerning the cogency of audiological recommendations.

With this handbook of advanced, multilayered strategies, I set out to work. I addressed all these resistance factors one by one. It was most likely that the audiologist explained to Norma that there may be initial discomfort when she started wearing the aids, but that it would be temporary. Her fine motor skills were sufficient for manipulating the hearing aid controls. Oral and clear written directions were repeatedly provided. Her children paid for the cost of the hearing aids in full.

We tried various methods of addressing her denial of hearing loss, i.e., by saying "it's normal for older people to not hear well," "the world isn't mumbling all of a sudden," and "it's not your fault." We discussed on how "it takes a strong person to use assistive devices" (borrowed from the Perdue chicken commercial "it takes a strong man to make a tender chicken"). When addressing possible stigma, I asked Joan to make lists of notable people who wore hearing aids, such as Ronald Reagan. We gave her previews of various social events in which she could participate. We regularly reminded her that "You have a whole life out there that you're missing—bingo, the bridge club, etc."

Joan and Marty even bribed her. (In psychology literature, this is called positive reinforcement.) For every week she wore her hearing aids, she would be taken out for a porterhouse steak, her favorite meal.

Norma, in turn, would reassure us that she appreciated— as she put it—our "kind efforts" and added that she also liked her audiologist and doctor: "They spend enough time with me and they're very nice people." At Christmas, she even sent us all cards and chocolates.

Despite our persistent and clever efforts, however, it was all to no avail.

"Why won't you wear them?" echoed her children.

"Please don't worry about me. I'll be fine."

"You have to wear them! We bought them! We paid for them! They will help you hear! Why won't you wear them? Why? Why?"

We had come full circle back to our first session, almost two months previously.

It was time for me to intervene from a different position to shift the balance of power. Whereas I had spent most of my efforts allying with the intentions of the family and professional network, here was an opportunity to definitively lobby in behalf of Norma. I looked directly at Joan and Marty and, in a much slower pace, asserted that "You know, both of you—and all of us—have good intentions, but Norma does have the right to say 'No.'"

My intervention worked. Norma immediately leaned forward in her chair, looked at her children, and smiled devilishly: "I remember when you two wouldn't eat your vegetables. What a fuss you used to make!"

"Mom, we're not hear to talk about vegetables. Now will you listen to reason and—"

"What kind of vegetables did they hate?" I asked Norma. It was important to continue upsetting the balance of power.

"Brussels sprouts. Gawd, how they would carry on!" she retorted.

"Ugh. I don't blame them," I said, at the same time protecting my alliance with Joan and Marty. "Especially the kind that's soaked in butter, all soft and mushy. Yech, I can't tell you how many times my dad and I fought about that, but they really are good for you: make you big and strong."

"Now Dr. Harvey," the children echoed, "about our mom, we think she just needs to accept her hearing loss and get on with her life. If we can just—"

"Why didn't you eat your brussels sprouts?" I inquired.

Dead silence. Then laughter; perhaps they thought I was kidding, but my expression indicated that I was not. "Didn't you know they were good for you?"

"C'mon doctor, you know we're not here to—"

"Vitamin D, 500 mg; Vitamin A, 352 mg; Vitamin B6, 343 mg. . . ." I continued to list the vitamins that brussels sprouts contained. The list took at least three minutes. (It was a total fabrication as I had no idea what those disgusting things contained, but at least to me, my vitamin analysis was impressive.)

Norma also seemed to enjoy the pedagogical discourse. As I ended, she lunged forward in her seat for the first time, and, also for the first time, her children leaned back. Now it was her turn: "And don't forget how good they are for your bones, your heart, lungs, liver, your spleen, your skin, . . ."

She, too, began a long list of benefits, probably also fabricated. She ended her retribution with "So, why won't you eat them? Why? Why?"

"Now, Mom, you know we're not here to talk about—"

"Don't you talk back to your mamma young man! Answer me!" Her nose flared and her face became flushed.

"Mom, we're grown children, you can't tell us to eat our vegetables anymore. Now please, will you—we all love you."

At this juncture, I began searching through my file cabinet. "Ah, here it is! An article on 'The Relationship between Management of Presbycusis and Ingestion of Brussels Sprouts by the Offspring: A Case Study.' Now let me just see what it says. Give me a minute."

The three of them sat, somewhat stupefied, watching me thumb through four or so pages. Even Norma thought I went off my rocker. The article was actually about "Decorating Your Office" but it would have to do.

"Well, it does seem that there may be some relationship between you two [Marty and Joan] eating your brussels sprouts and you [Norma] trying hearing aids, but it seems that more research is needed."

Again silence. This time punctuated by smirking. Joan asked Marty, "Where did we find this doctor? We should never have trusted the yellow pages."

"I agree," echoed Marty. "Besides, this doctor was your idea."

"It was not," Joan quipped.

"Was too."

"Was not."

"Was too."

"My god, what have I done?" I asked. I put down the article.

Everyone was getting a good chuckle out of this exchange. Although Norma could not track the fast pace of the conversation, she obviously enjoyed it. More importantly, as she intermittently chided her children for not eating enough vegetables—particularly Joan who was in Norma's words "premenopausal"—she seemed more empowered. Norma was now on a more equal footing with her kids, whom she perceived as having bullied her into coming to my office, albeit with good intentions.

The children's attempts to persuade Norma to wear hearing aids were analogous to Norma's much earlier attempts to persuade them to eat brussels sprouts. However, forty-plus years ago, Norma was the grown-up parent with the responsibility and authority to mandate ingestion of that awful green, mushy mass to her young children; today there were no young children in the room and the conflict was arising because Norma was still intellectually and emotionally competent enough to make informed decisions about her life, including audiological treatment, regardless of the fact that her now-grown children took on some levels of responsibility for her care.

At the beginning of one session, I directly asked Norma to elaborate what her fears and anxieties were about wearing hearing aids. As if she had been waiting for me to finally ask that question, she immediately responded "I'm not ready for an undertaker." I thought she misread my lips so I asked the question again, but she had understood everything. For Norma, using assistive listening devices felt like using a cane, a walker, or a pacemaker; she associated them with helplessness and an endless series of doctors visits. She ultimately viewed them as one giant step toward her own death.

She did not know how to share that private terror with her physician, her children, or anyone else. Instead, in reaction to her physician's solace and advice—"You should get hearing aids, join some support groups, take lip-reading classes; think of others who are worse off, who have terminal illness, who have. . . ."—she would reply "You're right, that's what I need to do; it could be much worse, at least I still have residual hearing." With her children, she comforted them by saying things like "Oh come now, it was a very nice party, it was very thoughtful of you." Finally, with me—until this moment—she had typically responded with something like "Don't feel sorry for me; I don't need your patronizing attitude; I don't need your sympathy; I'm coping with it just fine, thank you." When she felt particularly vulnerable—perhaps on the heels of a new round of tests for unexplained physical pain—she would glibly remark "There will always be death and taxes."

Now, something had changed. She elaborated on her reference to an undertaker with a twist on death and taxes: "I'm never ready to pay Uncle Sam, and I'm not yet ready for death, not yet."

"Please help me understand what using hearing aids has to do with death?" I asked.

"I'm not yet ready to let go."

"Let go of what, your life?" I asked.

"No, that I decide how I live my life, with whom I live, why I live, what help I want, and what help I don't want. It's something you young people can't understand." She paused, looking one by one at Joan, Marty, and me. Her countenance had changed to an odd combination of scorn and compassion.

"Give your damn hearing aids to someone else!" she yelled. "It's my life, my decision, my choice!"

Silence permeated the room. Soon it was time to stop.

Norma's declaration seemed straight out of a book by Albert Camus written over twenty-five years ago. Throughout the entirety of *Happy Death,* the protagonist sits with a gun forever at his side, an omnipresent reminder that at any given moment it is his existential decision, and his alone, whether or not to live. To be alive is to decide.[3]

If I could somehow enter that story, should I try to grab the gun away from him? Wouldn't he then be better off? Suppose it inadvertently fired? Suppose he had a lapse of judgement and shot himself? Suppose he realized that he was missing thousands of opportunities by continually sitting there with the gun?

Norma would be "better off" with hearing aids; he would be "better off" without the gun. A silly comparison, I first thought, as—unlike guns—there is no potential lethality with the use or misuse of hearing aids. But what was common between Norma and that man was their tenacity, their vehement insistence on exercising their own authority over their own lives, particularly when their decisions affronted a culture, family, doctors, etc., all of whom—albeit for benevolent purposes—were intent on abdicating their authority. In Norma's case, that benevolent or therapeutic goal was framed as "increasing patient adherence to audiologic recommendations."

My job now was to honor Norma as the teacher, to ask her to help me understand what was behind her decisions: how she experienced her acts of deciding in the context of her finite life. Although I must admit that, in some ways, it felt good to be included in the "you young people" category, I dreaded the next meeting. I was blown away by Norma's disclosure. The good and bad news was that she was finally talking openly about not yet being ready for death. (Isn't this what I had hoped for?) It was a subject that made eating brussels sprouts seem blissful.

Marty and Joan must have felt the same way. The next meeting began with awkward small talk about the Boston traffic—"it's getting worse, don't you think?"

I cut in and asked Marty and Joan what they thought about their mother's association of her audiologist to an undertaker. Perhaps because they also did not know how to respond and felt anxious themselves, they listed standard platitudes for Norma: "Oh come now, you'll be around for a long time; don't think about what you can't change; now just stay healthy, follow your doctor's orders and. . . ."

Norma, feeling a bit more empowered, restated her earlier evaluation of us "naive young people." "All these doctors' visits, pills, tests, and hearing aids affect my life and affect my death. I don't think you all understand; I don't know if you want to understand."

Norma became the teacher for all of us. However, as she correctly observed, it was questionable whether we were willing and able to be educated. The previous battle for compliance was now being played out in reverse. We were locked in a stalemate. For several sessions, we skirted around the issues of choice, mortality, and what's good for you.

That changed when Marty appeared for one session with bruises on his forehead. He briefly mentioned that he had tripped over a broom and had fallen down the basement stairs. He ended with "But I'm okay" and motioned me to begin the session.

"You could have gotten killed," I replied.

"Yeah, but I'm alright. Just some swelling, that's all." He again made eye contact with me as a nonverbal request that I move on. Seeing no response, he took the lead and stole my usual opening line: "So who wants to start?"

"We already have," I retorted. A golden opportunity not to be missed. "Would you be willing to play back when you fell down the stairs?"

"No thank you, Doc, once is enough!"

"No, I mean here, now—where it's safe." I explained my request to Marty asking that he walk us though in slow motion what he was thinking and feeling as he fell to the basement floor. "Did you see your death? Did you see your life flash by you? Did you try to bargain with God? What did you experience?"

Although his fall lasted only seconds, Marty confirmed—after some prodding by Norma and me (at this juncture, she and I were in sync)—that he nevertheless did simultaneously experience a long series of inner events and dialogues.

> "I saw myself lying on the cement floor bleeding to death. 'So this is how I would die,' I remember thinking.'But if for some reason I miraculously do not die, I'll spend more time with my kids and tell them how proud I am of them, how much I love them, how I'd do anything for them. I would take more time to breathe, not run in circles so much, not work so hard, and I would go to church. Please God, don't let me die now, please.'"

Marty's eyes were closed, his teeth were clenched, and both hands were clasped tight, as if holding onto to something for dear life.

"Death is a very scary thing." My meager contribution. By this time, my hands were clenched too.

An odd but serene silence now enveloped the room. No more battles. No more talk of vegetables. Something had happened, but exactly what I did not know.

Norma, and now Marty, knew. Norma broke the long silence by taking Marty's hand: "I'm glad you're okay; you could have been killed." A long pause. "I also know what's it's like to see death, but I won't die now. Later, but not now."

Teshuva

In the Midrash, an ancient Hebrew literary form, there is a story of Abraham exploring a cave. To his surprise, he found his own burial site. However, rather than flee from it, he remained and meditated at the site, and, like Marty, he found himself rehearsing his own death. Rabbi Lawrence Kushner described this process of Teshuva as "reexperiencing the Nothingness from whence we have come. . . . You cannot be reborn until you are willing to die. . . . The creation and maintenance of being require a kind of rhythmic moving out from and a returning to the point of beginning."[4]

Perhaps the Catholic equivalent of Teshuva is Lent. On Ash Wednesday, the priest says, "Remember you are dust and to dust you will return." Some sects of Buddhism refer to the transcendent state of nothingness as the satori experience.

Complicated words. Some things just have to be experienced to be understood; words are inadequate. (I guess that's what my dad meant when he would say "you'll understand when you grow up.")

Marty now understood; he had "grown up." His falling down the basement stairs catalyzed him to rehearse his death—perform Teshuva. It was his journey to the "Nothingness through which his consciousness was transformed."[5] It was also the same journey that Norma had begun, in part, catalyzed by the subject of hearing aids.

It was what she had been trying to tell us all along.

From then on our meetings would never be the same. Rather than each of us figuring out our strategies for the next battle, we gradually realized that much more was at stake. We became collaborators on a project of understanding the multilevel psychological, family, and spiritual dimensions of deafness and old age, all originally catalyzed by a visit to an audiologist. All of us adopted a stance of curiosity. Instead of being consumed by "why don't you" or "you should," we began to wonder aloud "what you feel when you . . ." or to ask another to "tell me what it's like to. . . ."

We met for three more months, a total of six months. Although Norma was wearing her hearing aids more often than not, it no longer consumed our discussions. We would occasionally reminisce about our earlier sessions when Norma would make what seemed like non sequiturs, i.e., interrupting a heated exchange by "I wonder what's happen on 'Wheel of Fortune'?" Now we were able to understand these subtle and other more overt gestures as her way of demarcating her sense of self from the prevailing opinions of her family and provider network. It was her way of establishing her authority.

———

An odd paradox: It is often harder to do something good for yourself when so many others are trying to convince you. You are never sure who the act benefits, yourself or others. More technically speaking, the boundaries between self and others become blurred. As Norma put it during the early days of our visits, "If I were to give in and put on those damn hearing aids, I may as well just lay down and die."

Death, however, does not have to be toxic. For Norma, the privacy of her associating the audiologist with an undertaker—her rehearsing her death in the absence of public validation or of spiritual support—rendered her hearing aids toxic. It compelled her to flee from the world, to protect her sense of self by opposing others, even when her opposition deprived her of opportunities. In the confines of her private death imagery, to capitulate to the wishes of others would have meant to die an inner, lonely death.

In contrast, as Norma publicized her death imagery to her family and felt an empathic connection with Marty through his own death rehearsal, she no longer felt alone. She felt validated in relation to a significant another. Consequently, she did not experience the loss of self by following doctors' orders. Making her death public had rendered it nontoxic.

I often marvel at how and why it was that soon after Norma rehearsed her death that Marty followed suit. I cannot help but wonder if this is what Psychiatrist Carl Jung meant by "synchronicity" or, in the concept's popular form, the "First Principle" in the best seller *Celestine Prophesy:* those apparent coincidences that are not really coincidences at all.[6]

After we had ended our meetings, I received cards from Norma, particularly around the holidays. She confirmed that she was doing fine and that she was making her children happy by wearing "those damn things [hearing aids]." Virtually all of her notes ended with a reminder for me to eat my vegetables.

I also occasionally got cards from Joan or Marty. They typically acknowledged that Norma was doing well but emphasized that "there must be a better way instead of us having to eat brussels sprouts." Apparently, Norma had insisted that they routinely eat that delicacy together and, in turn, she would wear her hearing aids. On occasion, Norma admitted to them that the hearing aids were helpful.

About five years ago, I received a letter from Joan saying that Norma had died peacefully in her sleep.

Old people still scare me, but perhaps a little bit less. I now realize the obvious that I am scared of my own aging. Now at the age of forty-five, I sometimes complain to others that I feel old, and, to my chagrin, I still get the same compassionate yet dismissive smirks that I remember getting at the age of thirty. A friend, age fifty-eight, says that I will feel differently "later."

What does he mean? Maybe, among other things, that not only do I now understand Norma in a different way than I did fifteen years ago, but also I will continue to understand her differently as I experience my own aging. I may have deeper insights into how I hopefully helped her and how she definitely helped me.

I am tempted to say that every time I eat brussels sprouts, I think of Norma, but as an adult, I never go near them—and never will. I do often think of her, however, when I have "family discussions" with my own kids about the virtues of doing one of several "you shoulds," such as eating vegetables. I have deep compassion for Joan, Marty, and health-care professionals for how we work hard at giving what we think is sound advice.

How helpless, pissed off, and self-righteous I feel when my kids look me square in the eyes and assert their voluminous "NO!" Then I lecture them on all the reasons why, and they lecture me on all the reasons why not. Most of the time, one of us begrudgingly gives in only to plan more advanced strategies for the next battle.

Every once in a while, often for only an instant, I am touched with a realization that our dialogue is part of a larger and more complex drama involving issues of autonomy, dependency, self-esteem, and love, and then, whether I win the battle doesn't seem quite so important anymore.

Notes

1. Erikson, E. H. (1968). *Identity, youth and crises*. New York: Norton.

2. Berezin, M.A., Liptzin, B., & Salzman, C.(1988). The elderly person. In *The new harvard guide to psychiatry*. Cambridge, MA: The Belknap Press.

3. Camus, A. (1972). *Happy death*. New York: Vintage International.

4. Kushner, L. (1981). *The river of light: Spirituality, Judaism, and consciousness*. Woodstock, VT: Jewish Lights Publishing.

5. Kushner, *River of light*.

6. Redfield, J. (1994). *The celestine prophecy: An adventure*. New York: Warner.

CHAPTER SEVEN

Tinnitus No More: Aspen Here I Come!

I met Jason just hours after a true-to-form Boston nor'easter. The howling wind had echoed through my office and ravaged the meager landscaping outside, but now everything was peaceful and serine. Not so for Jason, however, who had suffered from tinnitus since his mid-twenties. He was now forty-two years old.

One definition of tinnitus is "a sensation of sound heard in the head and ears when no corresponding outside sound is present."[1] Jason's description, however, is more poignant: "it feels like air-raid sirens pounding against my skull; other times its like water rushing back and forth and then like bells ringing or stones rubbing together." Tinnitus is experienced by as many as 50 million Americans and in many cases is accompanied by hearing loss. The incidence of tinnitus in the population seen in audiology clinics has been estimated to be as high as seventy-five percent![2] Tinnitus can result from a variety of causes, including damage or abnormalities anywhere along the auditory pathway, exposure to loud noise, ototoxic medications, or hypertension.[3] However, in Jason's case—as for most people—the cause of the tinnitus was unknown.

In anticipation of my questions, Jason dutifully produced an organized listing of all the specialists he had ever seen. It would be necessary to inquire in detail about their individual contributions to figure out how I might be of assistance. He clearly had undergone this initial interview ritual many times, and judging by his listlessness, he seemed resigned to many more repetitions in the future.

Jason told me that he had first mentioned to his internist being bothered by "water rushing around" in his head well over fifteen years ago. After an initial physical examination proved inconclusive, the doctor made a referral to an otolaryngologist, an ear nose and throat doctor (ENT). She ruled out more serious medical conditions and recommended audiological treatment.

However, it was ten years later when Jason finally made it to the audiologist's office. He recounted that the initial doctor's appointment took away the sense of urgency. In his words, "I was relieved that at least I didn't have some kind of brain tumor. Besides, the noises weren't bad at that time. I could live with it. I hoped that eating better and exercising more would make it would go away."

Instead, the tinnitus got worse. So at the age of thirty-eight, Jason took the next step and visited an audiologist whom he had heard lecture about "ringing in the ears." In addition to confirming tinnitus, the evaluation revealed nerve damage to the inner ear resulting in a mild-to-moderate hearing loss. Although additional diagnosis shook Jason up a bit, he was not totally surprised by it. As he recounted, "I had been asking the world to repeat things more and more over the past few years."

The audiologist recommended binaural hearing aids with a masking device, a small noise generator which fits into a hearing aid. She had explained to Jason that introducing an external sound frequently masks the tinnitus sound and provides relief, a process known as "residual inhibition."

Jason was enthusiastic about the treatment and the theory behind it. Within a few days, he purchased the hearing aids and masking device, but his momentum did not stop there. He did his own research and downloaded articles from the Internet describing the relationship between tinnitus and Temporomandibular Joint Dysfunction (TMJ), a misalignment of the jaw. He recognized his symptoms as characteristic of TMJ: he ground his teeth at night, heard popping noises when opening his mouth quickly, and experienced intermittent pain around his jaw.

So Jason immediately scheduled an appointment with a dentist who specialized in treating Temporomandibular Joint Dysfunction. The dentist confirmed the diagnosis and informed him that many people with tinnitus also have TMJ. He recommended facial exercises and coached him on specific sleeping positions that would minimize stress to his jaw. Jason recalled feeling proud of himself for his self-diagnosis and his active participation in his own recovery.

In my office, however, he did not seem proud or optimistic. Rather, I could sense the fatigue and despair in his voice and drooped eyes. He shook his head and sighed, as if to mark the end of his duty to catch me up. His countenance also forewarned me of his final comment: "Nothing so far has helped."

Now it was my turn. "You must feel helpless and desperate," I offered.

For an instant, I feared his response: perhaps something like "now that's a brilliant deduction, doc; where did you go to school?" This imagined rebuttal from Jason was my own internal "noise" about not being helpful enough quickly enough. It represented the part of me that, perhaps like Jason, was impatient to find a cure. Rather than ridicule my poo-pooing of the obvious, however, he visibly relaxed in his seat, exhaled deeply, and said "Boy, you got that right." For now, affirming Jason's experience was enough. He felt understood.

Affirming his despair also paradoxically seemed to give him vitality. He said, "But I'm not through; I don't like to give up!" He inhaled deeply as if to energize himself for the next series of hurdles which, in fact, he had already scheduled. More appointments, more initial interviews, more catching up doctors, and more tests. Jason provided me with the names of several neurologists and psychiatrists from whom he had recently sought consultation. He was also in the process of scheduling appointments with a nutritionist and an acupuncturist, and he had just joined a health club.

Jason's next question to me was his bottom line for our visit: "Do you think psychotherapy can help?"

I nodded my head, explaining how stress management training, in particular, may be effective in tinnitus symptom reduction. The severity of virtually every physical and psychological ailment is related to the level of stress: the worse the stress, the worse the ailment. We discussed in detail how tinnitus is one of many physical disorders that cause the psychological experience of pain. Therefore, our goal would be to reduce his pain by using various pain-management techniques.[4] Taking ownership of his tinnitus would be his first step toward gaining control over it.

In addition, we agreed on the importance of me helping him coordinate and make sense out of the multidisciplinary recommendations that continued to dominate his life. As author Thomas Mann advised, over seventy years ago, "Order and simplification are the first steps toward mastery of a subject—the actual enemy is the unknown."[5] Jason needed to understand and organize not only his internal experience, but also what had become overwhelming hordes of helpers.

Jason smiled and made eye contact with me. "That sounds good." His auditory reference was an interesting play on words, given that his experience of "bad sounds" brought him to my office. We made eight weekly appoint-ments and agreed to evaluate how our work was going after two months.

Documenting the Baseline Severity

The first step with Jason would be to distinguish two differ-ent but interrelated concepts: his sensation and his distress. "Tinnitus sensation" refers to its physical components, for example, loudness, pitch, pressure, and other physical at-tributes. "Tinnitus distress" refers to how one perceives or experiences the tinnitus symptoms, for example, relief, hopefulness, frustration, anxiety, anger, and so on.

These two factors of pain may be experienced quite dif-ferently. In the case of tinnitus, some people hear very loud, intrusive clanging in their ears that warrants a high tinnitus sensation rating. However, they may not be equally as dis-tressed by it. Conversely, others experience very mild sensa-tions of tinnitus but rate their distress as very high.

I asked Jason to give an overall rating for his tinnitus sensation and distress, on a scale from one to ten, with ten as the most severe. Without hesitation, he rated both as "at least a nine." He elaborated that "it's real loud [sensation] and bothers me unbearably [distress]."

It has been my experience that people frequently visual-ize elaborate scenes or stories that incorporate the acoustic intrusions of tinnitus and that vary, depending on the level of sensation and distress. I inquired about Jason's imagery and any drama that may happen in his head. He pondered, perhaps because he was dumfounded by the question itself or because he had never before been given the opportunity to answer it. It turned out to be the latter. After only a few seconds of reflection, he replied "Sure, I can tell you ex-actly what I imagine happening inside of me; I've thought about it many times. A ton of bricks keeps falling on a pile of church bells. Sometimes I imagine that someone is throwing them down—maybe Hercules—so hard that the shock waves blast against my skull and that the heat discharge shoots out against my face and head. Other times, it feels like my brain is gurgling, like when I visited Yellowstone [National Park] and saw the bubbles coming up from the earth. Other times, it's like someone's mowing the lawn with a loud lawn mower, and sometimes it hits a rock and goes 'clunk.'"

Jason was clearly in a lot of pain.

I wondered whether his imagery and the levels of his sensation and distress varied during the day. Nighttime? Before and after meals? Upon waking up? With certain medications? Foods? After certain events? I suggested that Jason keep a tinnitus diary, which is standard practice in pain management programs. He agreed to record the following information at least three times daily: the situation in which he experienced tinnitus; a rating of the sensation; a description of the sensation; a rating of his distress; a description of his distress; and a description of the actions that he took to relieve his pain.

At first, Jason reacted with a sigh. I imagined that he felt burdened by more work and more record keeping. Upon my inquiry, he confirmed my hunch, but added "I'm afraid it will make me notice my tinnitus more."

"Do you fear that it will get worse?" I asked.

He quickly shook his head. "God no, it can't get much worse. I just won't be able to pretend it's not there," he replied.

Jason was hanging on to ways he could still deny many of the nuances of his tinnitus experience—those he could still control. Emphasizing his active control would be important to allay his fears about an imminent relapse.

"It sounds like you had already chosen to stop pretending that your tinnitus wasn't there when you decided to see the audiologist four years ago. It hasn't gotten worse, has it?"

He shook his head.

"You'll continue to make decisions all along the way." I added.

Once reassured, he asked me for more details on recording the data.

The purpose of his keeping a diary was partially for evaluation. It would help elucidate many more fluctuations of his pain that he had previously denied—had "pretended weren't there." But perhaps more importantly, it was an essential therapeutic intervention. Keeping a diary would give him a sense of empowerment—in his words, of "doing something about it." This was one of his primary coping mechanisms that had served him well.

He came in the following week, proudly carrying a leather-bound book that he had bought "on sale." Jason had taken the time to etch "Tinnitus Diary" on the cover in beautiful calligraphy. Similarly, his diary entries were impeccably organized and detailed. This ritual had clearly given him a sense of mastery. Diagnostically, it became apparent that both his tinnitus sensation and distress were typically a seven upon awakening in the morning. All other times and situations typically received sensation and distress ratings of nine. He got no relief!

Hypnosis

Clinical hypnosis is often used in the treatment of tinnitus as one of a variety of multimodal stress reduction approaches. Like meditation or biofeedback, it is a very powerful method of helping one achieve a deep state of relaxation and of changing specific thoughts or feelings. Jason was enthusiastic about using hypnosis, adding that he had already read a lot about it. I gave him my standard opening speech, essentially to dispel common myths about hypnosis which are conveyed through stage shows, i.e., that it makes people do things against their will or turns people into chickens.

He forced a rare smile. I continued the joke, saying that he should be concerned only if he starts laying eggs. He replied that I would be the first to know.

To my relief, Jason was very hypnotizable.* Within only a couple of sessions, he was able to achieve a deep hypnotic trance. He reported a profound sense of relaxation and detachment while keeping his eyes open, and he was able to verbalize his internal experiences to me. In this state, although his tinnitus sensation ratings remained stable at eight or nine, he reported that they bothered him less, warranting a distress severity rating of only four or five.

After the hypnotic session, Jason's reaction was cautious optimism, but he clearly was impressed. I was also confident we were on the right path.

However, at other times under hypnosis, a paradoxical effect occurred. Although Jason perceived the noises as softer (warranting a sensation rating of six), he was more bothered by them. His tinnitus distress ratings increased to ten! The hypnotic trance had heightened his awareness of the auditory intrusions. Although I assured him that, from my experience, this paradoxical effect sometimes occurs during states of deep relaxation or meditation, we were both disappointed. How we had hoped for a quick cure!

However, we had other tools at our disposal. We could use hypnosis not only to achieve relaxation, but also to change Jason's internal imagery and narrative with respect to the bricks and church bells. Although changing one's accompanying thoughts and feelings does not necessarily change the objective course of tinnitus, it can certainly change one's experience of its severity, the distress level. Pain, after all, is a psychological phenomenon which is only in part dependent on a physical lesion.

---

*Hypnosis is effective with both deaf and hearing people. Profoundly deaf people are asked to keep their eyes open.

Jason and I had agreed earlier that I would use hypnotic suggestion to replace his rather harsh, self-punitive imagery and narrative with something more benign. Easier said than done. His internal drama that began with "a ton of bricks falling on church bells" was not a result of random chance. The imagery represented a kind of psychic equivalent of the tinnitus sounds. Jason, albeit unconsciously, incorporated the auditory intrusions from his tinnitus into a narrative, a story; he made the sounds become part of his internal drama.

As an illustration of this process, there was a man who had a dream about swimming down a waterfall, only to realize later that he had left his shower on all night. The shower appeared in his dream as a waterfall. Similarly, Jason's tinnitus appeared in his imagery as falling bricks. For a variety of reasons—many of which remain mysterious—these particular images had credibility for the dreamer and for Jason. Each perceived the waterfall and the bricks as being similar enough to the shower and the tinnitus, respectively, to pass a sort of "unconscious audition" and become symbols in their internal drama.

Jason's internal drama contained sounds, images, and feelings. In more technical jargon, the symbolic representations of his tinnitus appeared in his narrative via the auditory, visual, and kinesthetic modalities.[6]

1. **Auditory Modality**

   "church bells"; "loud lawn mower"; "clunk."

2. **Visual Modality**

   "Hercules throwing bricks"; "saw the bubbles coming up from the earth"; "someone's mowing the lawn."

3. **Kinesthetic Modality**

   Heat: "heat discharge shoots out against my face and head."

Pressure: "a ton of bricks keep falling so hard"; "shock waves blast against my skull"; "my brain is gurgling."

The "replacement drama" would have to offer alternative sensations via these three modalities with equal credibility.* Moreover, the replacement drama must be both coherent and meaningful to Jason. Otherwise, why would he give up the original one? Painful as it was, at least it was familiar and held meaning for him.

For a substitute auditory sensation, we decided on the sound of ocean waves, as it relaxed him and represented, in his words, "a spiritual center." In addition, as Jason and I were both fans of the Beatles, we selected the music build-up at the end of "A Day in the Life" from the Sergeant Pepper album (our favorite), specifically focussing on the part of the song which had the same pitch and intensity as his tinnitus.

For substitute visual sensations, we chose a scene from his all-time favorite vacation spot: a sunrise over the majestic mountains of Aspen, Colorado.

His original internal drama also contained heat and pressure kinesthetic reactions that also needed to be replaced. For heat, we chose the comfort and warmth of bathing in a hot tub, again derived from his previous Aspen vacations. For pressure, we embellished the sensation of warmth with "the gentle gurgling and pulsating of the hot tub jets."

We were finally ready to replace his original drama under hypnosis. When he reached a deep trance state, I suggested to him "As you continue to go deeper and deeper into the trance, you once again see Hercules throwing

---

*This technique is derived from neuro-linguistic programming, well known to practitioners of hypnosis. The reader is referred to Bandler and Grinder.

bricks on church bells, you feel the heat, and you hear the noises, but this time, it begins to change as you go deeper into a relaxing, soothing trance. You see yourself bathing in an outdoor hot tub in Aspen. Your favorite spot. It feels good to enjoy the warmth of the water against your skin, the comfort, warmer and more comfortable than it was a minute ago. The rhythmic sound of the ocean, the waves, in and out, in and out (I timed this with his breathing). In the distance, behold the music (I do my best to imitate the tune). It's a good feeling to allow yourself to relax, a good feeling, in and out, feel the warmth, the bubbles, the gentle gurgling and pulsating of the hot tub jets, the comfort. . . ."

I repeated this drama again and again for well over a half-hour. Jason's face beamed while he—at least psychologically—was in the hot tub enjoying the more benign auditory, visual, and kinesthetic experiences. Of greater importance, upon waking up from the hypnotic trance, he reported a tinnitus distress rating of only three. We were both exuberant!

During the next several sessions, we routinely revisited Aspen and enjoyed the sounds, views, and feelings that it had to offer. When he was hypnotized, he would fairly consistently report tinnitus distress ratings of only between three and five, a far cry from his typical ratings of seven to nine. We also shared a bit of nostalgia and creativity together, as we occasionally altered the musical part of the imagery, substituting a Pink Floyd song in place of the Beatles. Other times, we chose Jimi Hendrix.

Jason easily learned to hypnotize himself at home and was proud of his new-found skill to change his internal drama while incorporating his unremitting tinnitus sounds. We discussed the advantages of using a variety of other relaxation and meditation tools, such as John Kabat-Zinn's "mindfulness meditation."[7] This is a very helpful technique that encourages one to remain passively focused on the pain—to allow oneself simply to observe the pain and the resulting feelings without becoming consumed by them.

Through these eclectic approaches, Jason experienced success. Falling bricks became crashing ocean waves; church bells became melodies; heat discharges became the hot tub. He could go into a trance state almost at will in a variety of situations, whether hanging out at home, on his Nordic Trac, or at a restaurant. He mentioned in passing that he even took an imaginary trip to Aspen while he and his partner made love.

In a trance state, his typical tinnitus sensation ratings dropped to six, and his distress ratings dropped to four! As he continued to practice self-hypnosis, to conduct his own research, and to schedule appointments with other professionals, he felt renewed hope and confidence. He enjoyed demonstrating his self-advocacy skills and kept himself busy investigating the credentials of various neurologists, psychiatrists, nutritional consultants, and acupuncturists. He joined the American Tinnitus Association. Jason was on a roll.

I wish this story could end here, perhaps with "and he lived happily ever after," but for reasons unknown, Jason's improvement was elusive and transitory. After hours or sometimes a day of a relatively low level of tinnitus sensation and distress, his tinnitus would return in full force with a demonic wrath. There were no new stresses in his life and no changes in his health. It was as if the tinnitus itself sentenced him to suffer for having enjoyed even a brief respite. Jason provided this anthropomorphic interpretation, now viewing the tinnitus, at best, as an unwelcome guest, at worst, as "an executioner." We were dumbfounded.

Private torture. There were times when Jason's tinnitus became so unbearable that he entertained thoughts of suicide. "With death there would at least be peace and quiet." It was safer to remain in the melancholy abyss than to climb out and then be pulled back in.

Jason and I requested psychiatric consultation for medication, as he became increasingly depressed and was not sleeping well. Severe depression for people with tinnitus is not unusual. It stems from the severity of the head noise itself, sleep loss and, equally as important but often unrecognized, the loneliness of feeling that, in Jason's words, "nobody understands and, even worse, they think I'm overreacting." His best friend's well-meaning advice was to "ignore it." He might as well have asked Jason to spread his wings and fly.

The psychiatrist immediately confirmed that Jason had common symptoms of depression. Whether tinnitus caused some or all of these symptoms was unknown. In any event, the treatment was to prescribe a common antidepressant, Nortriptyline (Pamelor).[8] After a trial period of a month with no appreciable effect, the medication was changed to another antidepressant, Fluoxetine (Prozac).* In addition, the psychiatrist prescribed Clonazapam (Klonopin), an anti-anxiety medication to hopefully reduce his stress and therefore his tinnitus sensations and/or distress.

Jason reported that the medications helped "take the edge off" his depression but he did not notice any appreciable change in his tinnitus levels. To this day, he continues to take these medications.

Jason also visited an allergist. Allergic reactions often affect the functioning of the middle ear, which may cause tinnitus. The doctor prescribed an over-the-counter antihistamine, Chlortrimeton, to treat possible eustachian tube and middle ear blockage. Since it did not help Jason's tinnitus and it caused fatigue, the doctor then prescribed a nonsedative antihistamine, Terfenadine (Seldane). However, after a couple of months with no results, Jason discontinued this medication.

---

*Some tricyclic antidepressants appear to help tinnitus but researchers are unsure why.

Acupuncture was his next stop. He went for three months. No results. His internist gave him a diuretic, Furosemide (Lasix), that specifically exerts its effect on the kidney and the inner ear. No results. Then an Herbology consult. No results. Then a nutritional consultation. No results. Then a thorough neurological workup, complete with a CT scan. He checked out as normal.

It was time for Jason and I to reevaluate our goals. For two months, we had labored to achieve a narrowly defined objective: to decrease his tinnitus sensation or at least his distress. Although he did experience periods of improvement, these times became fraught with anxiety. It meant succumbing to renewed hopes and optimism that inevitably permeated his self-protective wall of cynicism, and then the crash when his hopes were maliciously shattered. Soothing hot tubs in Aspen would soon become superimposed with bricks crashing into church bells.

Sometimes his rage would break through. He would pound his fist on the table, curse, and kick furniture clear across the room! Then the irony of such outburst became apparent. As Jason put it, "I can't get so mad. Stress makes my tinnitus worse!"

His stress and despair were contagious. I, too, somehow felt betrayed and cheated—like we had both gotten a raw deal. After all, we had been working hard. Jason could not have been more conscientious about practicing new skills, requesting consults and record-keeping. I found myself frequently thinking about him during the week, wondering how he was doing. I read everything I could get my hands on about treating tinnitus. Jason deserved more success.

We got some solace by reminding ourselves how little is understood about this disorder. In part, we were obliged to honor our commitment to be honest and open about treatment progress. Most of all, however, we acknowledged to each other our disappointment. We could not hide our feelings, even if we tried.

If you cannot rid yourself of a burden, what do you do with it?

Jason and I continued to meet, now biweekly, both to continue hypnotherapy and to check in. We continually shifted our focus back and forth between attempting to reduce his tinnitus and accept it as one of the many blemishes of his life. To accept what you simultaneously attempt to change. A paradox to be sure, but not an uncommon one.

During the checking in part of our discussions, we gradually found ourselves departing from our narrow focus on his tinnitus symptoms. Instead, we chatted about his life, his hobbies, his relationships, and his upbringing. Any subject was deemed worthy of discussion and examination. He told me how his earlier life had been idyllic, "like a fairy tale." He was popular, and had always done well in school. In his words, "everything always came easy for me."

I told Jason a story about a man who spent several years and a lot of money designing and building his dream house. Ideal construction, floor plan, color scheme, location, etc. One day, however, a drunk neighbor banged on his door. The woman screamed at him that his house had caused her basement to flood and abruptly stormed away, only to return several days later. She would not listen to the city authorities who informed her that her claim was unfounded.

The man attempted to humor her, ignore her, and yell back at her, and when those strategies failed, he threatened her with legal action for harassment, but nothing worked. Even when she did not come for weeks, he would sit on his couch, staring out of his bay-view window, but not at the beautiful view. He continually stared at that woman's house. His dream had been blemished.

So maybe Jason would need to accept his tinnitus as unchangeable. We cannot always choose what burdens get placed on us. We cannot always choose our neighbors. Jason had diligently followed each and every suggestion of the various helpers that had dominated his life for over two decades. He exercised, meditated, did Yoga, kept nutritional charts, followed medication regimens, took vitamins, kept countless doctors' appointments, changed his eating and sleeping habits, recited daily positive affirmations, read self-help books, attended self-help seminars, had psychotherapy, kept a diary, and prayed to a higher power. Half-jokingly, he reportedly even repented for whatever past-life sins he may have committed by forgoing Heath Bar ice cream for a week.

Nothing had produced lasting results. I repeatedly thought of our first meeting when he recounted a long, frustrating history of treatment failures.

———

It is often difficult to categorize the results of psychotherapy as success or failure, triumph or defeat. At this writing, Jason and I meet approximately once a month. He still suffers from tinnitus, although he has more periods of respite. He goes to work the best he can but there are some days that he cannot concentrate long enough to be productive.

On his optimistic days, he reminds himself that he is not in as much distress as he once was (his distress ratings typically vary between five and eight), even when his tinnitus sensations are severe, and he is hopeful that a new drug or cure will "take care of the rest." On his pessimistic days, he finds himself trapped by the less severe but nevertheless debilitating noises. He frequently succumbs to despair.

Unfortunately, this chapter is not a tale of triumph with a happy ending. If by triumph, we mean removal of his tinnitus, then we half-failed, half-succeeded. What is the value of an intimate collaboration with hard work when it fails to achieve its intended results?

I will never forget one moment with Jason. We had been working together for about twenty sessions over two years.

It was mid-afternoon on a warm spring day—a blue sky, light breeze, and bright sunshine. I was looking forward to later taking a walk with my wife and our dog and barbecuing chicken on our new grill. I would then finish a book and watch an old Colombo rerun.

All that would have to wait. It was time for our meeting. Jason entered my office, looking as somber and defeated as he had during our initial visit. Today he was pessimistic. His world often did not contain serene walks, relaxation, and Colombo reruns. It remained frequently polluted by ringing bells and clunking noises, by falling bricks, and by despair. He told me all of this once again, as he had told it to me many times before.

At that moment, I found myself unable to offer any more suggestions, ideas, treatment options, or referrals. I was only able to say "I'm sorry you're still in so much pain." A déjà-vu to our first session. We had come a full circle.

Jason curled up in his seat, almost in the fetal position, as if suffocated by the weight of his own body; I was leaning toward him in my chair with tears cascading down. He, too, began to cry. After what seemed like an eternity, he reached over and clasped my hands, more and more tightly, more and more desperately. I embraced his hands also as tightly as I could until it was time to end.

It is difficult to describe the intensity of that eternal moment. Many hours afterward, I did take my walk, barbecue the chicken, read, and enjoy watching Colombo solve yet another unsolvable crime, but that moment came back to me throughout the evening. To this day, it remains forever etched in my mind. Sometimes I resent that unwelcome intrusion into my own internal drama. The memory is not a happy one. I could not help him purge his tinnitus, as he had requested.

Other times, though, I feel honored. Jason shared with me a part of his tormented world that he dared not show another soul. He allowed me to help him put words to it, to illuminate its complexity—to bear witness. Not only did Jason achieve a certain depth that was otherwise unachievable, but also our joint odyssey gave me a renewed awe and appreciation for the ecstatic and desolate duality of my own life. During these times, that moment is a welcome guest, one that I would never ask to leave.

At present, Jason and I are focussing on developing his coping skills with respect to his rage and despair which consume him when his tinnitus is severe. We talk a lot about expectations and ways of asking for emotional support from others. Once a "confirmed bachelor," he has begun to date. In between his bouts of—in his words—"internal bombing, scraping, pounding, hammering, pummeling, pulsating, and throbbing" he manages to have good days.

I hope and pray that Jason's suffering will have a happy ending. Are my prayers enough? Along with our continued hard work, it would have to be, at least for now.

Notes

1. Saunders, J. (1992). *Tinnitus: What is that noise in my head?* Auckland, New Zealand: Sandalwood Enterprises.

2. Tyler, R. S. (1997). Tinnitus: current theories and treatments. *The Hearing Journal,* 50(8), 10–19.

3. Saunders, *Tinnitus.*

4. Caudill, M. A. (1995). *Managing pain before it manages you.* New York: The Guilford Press.

5. Mann, T. (1924). The magic mountain. Quoted in Caudill, M. A. (1995). *Managing pain before it manages you.* New York: The Guilford Press.

6. Bandler, R., & Grinder, J. (1975). *Patterns of the hypnotic techniques of Milton H. Erickson, M.D.* (Vol. 1). Palo Alto, CA: Science and Behavior Books.

7. Kabat-Zinn, J. (1990). *Full catastrophe living: Using the wisdom of your body and mind to face stress, pain and illness.* New York: Delecorte Press.

8. Tabachnick, B. (1995). *Drugs and tinnitus relief.* Tinnitus Today, 20(1), 7–12.

CHAPTER EIGHT

Escaping the Dungeon of Oppression

I do not think of Ann as having a hearing loss. Although she became profoundly deaf at the age of two from spinal meningitis, she has cherished memories of a childhood filled with Deaf peers, Deaf community, and Deaf culture. "Where's my loss if I have no memory of being able to hear?" she would ask. Far from viewing herself as disabled or hearing-impaired, she identified herself as culturally Deaf. Although she was only twenty-eight years old, she was a respected member of various community organizations.

Ann's first question to me on the TTY before making an appointment was whether or not I sign. A typical and vital inquiry. American Sign Language was her primary means of expressing her thoughts and feelings with the depth and nuances that I take for granted with spoken English. She would later tell me that she found lip-reading to be a laborious, frustrating, and imperfect art. Same for speech.

Upon meeting Ann, we first exchanged name signs, a meeting ritual among culturally Deaf people, much like exchanges of names among hearing people. She signed ASL beautifully, almost in a poetic fashion. I was in awe of how she used so many linguistic nuances to articulate her thoughts and feelings and with such vividness and passion. It came as no surprise to learn that she was much sought after as a Sign Language mentor by hearing as well as Deaf people.

I, too, signed ASL and attempted to match her clarity and language style. Attempt as I did, I could not completely succeed. Although I have practiced ASL for over fifteen years, it is not my primary language. Ann, however, said that my signing was clear and that she understood me. "Not bad for a hearing person," she quipped. Like many culturally Deaf people, she added that she respected hearing people, in large part, on the basis of their signing skills.[1] I had apparently passed that test.

To say the obvious, a therapist and client must use the same language.* However, obvious as it may be, Deaf people have observed that many times hearing professionals do not even understand the issue of communication and its importance. As a result, there is a long history of Deaf people being misdiagnosed as retarded or as emotionally disturbed.[2] A hearing person's lack of sign language skills has long been recognized as the primary cause of damaging cross-cultural interactions and of the acrimony toward hearing people that can be harbored by Deaf people.[3]

I made sure to ask Ann to stop me when and if I was not clear in my signing, and we also agreed that I would do the same when and if I did not understand her. In the old days, I would routinely ask "Do you understand me?" but I was informed that my question was demeaning, albeit with good intentions, as it put the onus of responsibility for assuring adequate communication on the Deaf person. I now phrase my question as "Am I clear?"

---

*Although an interpreter can assist with communication, the addition of a third party affects the quality of the therapeutic relationship and may introduce discomfort about confidentiality. Direct communication is preferable.

Ann wanted to know a bit about my background and how I got involved in the field of deafness. An interesting question and also a common one for Deaf clients to ask of hearing therapists. Their query is frequently a polite form of "Will you—like those others—misdiagnose me as intellectually defective or disturbed? Do you help deaf people to feel superior, to dominate, colonize, or eradicate them?" Those others once proposed a eugenics movement which would have sterilized prospective Deaf mothers![4]

With Ann, it would be critically important to differentiate myself from "those others." I could do this best via self-disclosure about how and why I got involved in the field of deafness. I told her my own story of having been captivated by the beauty of ASL poetry. I also recounted with Ann those Deaf community leaders who had been my teachers of ASL and of Deaf culture.

She nodded her head with tentative approval. Ann was relieved that I was familiar with the Deaf community and that I knew many of its members quite well. However, she expressed some common concerns about confidentiality: "You're not going to gossip about me, are you?" I therefore outlined very carefully the parameters of how our dialogue would remain private.

I then asked her to tell me a bit about her background and how she thought I could help. She had attended a prominent residential school for the deaf, where she learned American Sign Language, and then Gallaudet University. With obvious pride, she recounted her active role in the Deaf President Now revolution when, in 1988, Deaf students demanded and won increased representation on campus.

In stark contrast, however, was her description of her family life. Ann told me that both of her parents were hearing and did not sign. With a deep sigh, she added that "they forced me to go to speech therapy so I would become more hearing, but it didn't work." With a blank, vacant stare, Ann also recalled how her parents could neither understand her speech nor her signs—and how she typically could not understand them.

It was a familiar scenario. Like many newcomers to the field of deafness, I was initially shocked to learn about the many experiences of conversational isolation within hearing families of origin, but gradually and insidiously, the stories of pain became routine—the norm. Perhaps like many Deaf people, I, too, coped by numbing-out with a blank, vacant stare.

Ann described in more detail how her parents had pathologized her deafness by "dragging me to a million doctors." She emphasized "I've always been happy being Deaf but all they have ever done is badger me about getting a cochlear implant!" Now with her fist clenched, she proclaimed how much "they oppressed me." She gritted her teeth as if poised for combat, but, perhaps ever so slightly, I also detected what may have been a welled-up tear, particularly when she recalled how her dad favored her hearing brother. There is a thin line between rage and despair.

Ann's outcry had pierced my protective wall of routinized expectations. I could numb-out no more.

She had experienced oppression not only within in her family, but also in various job environments. Like many Deaf people, she tolerated the "glass ceiling" of underemployment, subtle and overt discrimination, and inadequate, if any, interpreters. She recalled that "There was one interpreter who had barely taken any signing courses and couldn't even sign 'good morning' properly!" When Ann had spoken up about such inadequate accommodations, she was typically labeled a troublemaker and/or was fired.

Our meeting was half over. We had exchanged in-depth introductions, she had provided me with a poignant summary of her history, and we seemingly decided that we could work together. I wondered aloud why Ann wanted therapy at this particular time, because those reported incidents of oppression had been happening to her for some time.

She responded "I'm in a new job and have a hearing, male boss who doesn't care about deafness and who is very oppressive. I hate him! I want you to teach me how to play hearing politics with that bastard so he doesn't fire me." Her request was to the point, but it was not clear. Did she want me to coach her on how to be passive and complacent amidst injustice or was she requesting me to coach her on how to be assertive, to advocate for herself, to triumph over her boss—the enemy, the colonizer, the oppressor.

Alternatively, did she want me to serve, not as a coach but as a guide—a sort of psychological mirror—to help her learn about her own internal reactions to oppression? As a guide or mirror, I would help her maintain her personal dignity in the face of oppression. She would learn to differentiate when she was, in fact, being victimized from when she may subtly, perhaps out of habit, encourage others to victimize her. Finally, she would be better able to determine whether she was feeling overly threatened by innocent people because they somehow reminded her of other oppressors in her life.

Ann confirmed that she wanted both a political coach and a psychological mirror: "I want tips, suggestions, and techniques I can use with my boss, and I want a better understanding about how I deal with bastards like him."

I then asked her my usual question, "Why did you choose me as your therapist?" Her answer: "Because you're hearing. You're separate from the Deaf community. I won't see you all the time at social gatherings." Her answer did not surprise me. However, I was nevertheless bound to see her at Deaf community events because of my ongoing contact with the Deaf community, in part, to maintain my signing skills and my awareness of cultural issues. Thus, Ann and I agreed on mutually comfortable rules of conduct for unplanned contact outside the office. We would simply say "hello" to each other.

It was time to end our meeting. On the whole, I felt our dialogue had gone well and she requested several more appointments, but it also felt uneasy and unsettling. I sensed that she had left something unsaid, perhaps that I had put her off in some way, had signed ASL poorly, or an infinite number of other possibilities. She bid me a polite but terse goodbye. I quickly jotted down in my notes "rocky road ahead?" before beginning my next appointment.

We met again a week later. In negotiating a treatment contract with Ann, it was initially easier for me to say what I could not do than what I could do. I could not guarantee to protect her job at her company, and I could not rectify hearing peoples' views of Deaf people, including those of her boss. At a minimum, I made a private commitment not to oppress her. She had had enough of that from others. A noble goal, but in retrospect, a bit simplistic.

Per Ann's request, I began by suggesting tips on how to deal with her boss. As it turned out, he had just given her a written warning for "insubordinate behavior" and Ann naturally wanted to respond the right way. My advice included both modifications of the "count to ten" wisdom that many of our parents have imparted to us and methods of being direct. We talked a lot about the differences between what she termed "hearing culture wishy-washiness" and "Deaf culture bluntness." For several sessions, we role played various tactics and nonverbal behaviors with which she could respond to her boss.

During our discussions, Ann often switched between using American Sign Language and a sort of Pidgin Sign English without voice. I matched her communication mode, but she constantly tested whether I understood her signing, obviously fearing that I was only pretending to understand her. Most of the time, however, I followed her quite easily and continued to stop her whenever that was not the case. Although I was aware of becoming somewhat fatigued—maybe even mildly irritated—due to the constant testing, I quickly came to appreciate the impact of her long-standing experiences of not being understood.

As our meetings continued, I sensed that she was slowly trusting my assurances. I felt relieved. Soon our communication became the lesser of many rocks in the rocky road that I had tentatively predicted earlier. Ann regularly interrupted my coaching with angry accusations that I wanted her to become more hearing and that I secretly agreed with her boss. "How could you suggest that I do that?" became her frequent complaint. "Now you're sounding just like that bastard! You think he's right and don't even care how I feel!"

In typical conversation Ann would explain her constant experiences of feeling stuck and victimized at work. I would summarize her sentiments. She would acknowledge that I did understand. We would both feel like we were getting somewhere.

"So now what do I do?" she would plead.

"Let me suggest—"

"You think you know it all, don't you?" She would cut me off before I could complete my thought.

Variations of the conversation sequence occurred again and again for several meetings. During one such exchange, I attempted to avoid any semblance of giving her "hearing-based" suggestions by reflecting the challenge back on her in an effort to encourage her to problem solve: "No, I don't have the answer," I emphasized. "Let's list some options on what you could do."

"Tell me what you think I should do!" she scowled.

"I don't know. Let's figure it out together."

"You do know!"

"How can you be so sure?" I asked.

"You're hearing. My boss is hearing. My whole damn company is hearing!"

"So?"

We had reached an impasse, but I was intrigued by her reference to "you're hearing." Was Ann putting me in the role of a hearing authority figure who, perhaps like her parents and "whole damn company," deemed themselves as right and her as wrong? (She had told me earlier that she typically couldn't lip-read her parents—particularly when they were angry and critical of her—but "they looked smart.") I wondered whether I was the recipient of her wrath that belonged more to "those others"—most recently, her boss.

Did I, in fact, agree with her boss? After all, Ann appeared to set up situations that would result in him reprimanding her, for example, by purposely not following his instructions on specific projects. She often would not show up for important department meetings nor would she respond to her boss's requests for an explanation. If her demeanor with me was any indication, her approach at work was anything but affiliative. I often found myself wondering whether she scowled more at work than she did with me.

I reminded myself that it is an error to blame the victim. Those who are victimized by oppression are more sensitive to it than are the oppressors. Instead of seeing a world full of opportunities, they may see a world full of injustices and psychological "dungeons." Far from being paranoid, it is often an accurate reflection of reality. Oppression is a recurring ordeal for most every Deaf person, even if it is committed, in Psychologist Harlan Lane's words, with a mask of benevolence.[5]

I tried my best to validate Ann's world view and encouraged her to describe additional instances of when she was excluded at work. In the middle of describing an incident during which a co-worker asked if she wouldn't mind lip-reading part of a training seminar, she recalled some so-called "benevolent" advice her parents had received. Educators had advised her parents to make sure that she only lip-read and used speech. They were advised to punish her if she used any Sign Language. "It was supposed to be for my own good," she said with a sarcastic tone, "since they thought that I would rely on sign language as a crutch."

Ann's childhood plight reminded me of a poignant passage from a recent text entitled *A Journey Into the Deaf-World:* ". . . whatever the intentions of the hearing parents of a Deaf child, when they deprive that child of the opportunity [to learn sign language], it appears to many members of the Deaf-World as child abuse. The term used in the Deaf-World is communication violence, and most Deaf people have been victims of it in one form or another."[6]

How could Ann effectively address such communication violence at her present work place? We discussed how institutional change happens, using the Deaf President Now revolution as a prime example. I also brought up some tactics that other oppressed minority cultures have used, ranging from those of Mahatma Gandhi to those of Eleanor Roosevelt and Eldridge Cleaver and wondered aloud how, or if, she could modify them at her work place. We discussed polite yet assertive methods of requesting and/or demanding competent interpreters, note-takers, etc.

As before, however, she returned to venting about how her boss was "really an asshole." She refused to formulate any ways that she could help create positive change. Her signing became fast-paced and I had to ask her a few times to repeat herself. Not surprisingly, she then exploded. "God damn it, I'm tired of all you hearing people not getting it, not understanding me. C'mon get with it! I'm not signing it again! I'm tired of it, fed up!" Her indictments—which had been directed toward her boss—were now directed toward me.

"I'm not going to pretend to understand you when I don't," I pleaded. "What you're saying is too important for that."

More indictments followed. She then stood up, shot daggers at me with her eyes, and motioned to leave. "Work doesn't include me in conversations! The interpreter's sign language sucks! My boss is an asshole! Oppression! And you sit there so smug, trying to sign ASL, probably thinking about your hearing clients—how much you're looking forward to seeing them!"

Once she began discharging her rage at me, she did not want to stop. Certainly, this was not the time to justify my expressive signing ability nor to address the topic of other clients. It was a time to allow and encourage Ann to verbally confront a hearing authority figure without recrimination. She had never used this opportunity before and it was long overdue.

I simply remained seated with her and waited. Seeing no offensive reaction from me, she continued to unleash her fury. It continued for several minutes. After what seemed like a long while, her face softened a bit and became somber. Perspiration was streaming down her forehead. Her signing became a bit slower and smaller. She finally repeated what she had signed earlier. I replied that I understood.

It was time for me to bring up a long overdue subject: Ann and I needed to talk about our relationship. I asked her whether she viewed me as oppressive and abusive. After a long pause, she finally openly stated what she had hidden from herself and from me—what had been buried beneath her rage: "I need you to understand me, you know? Sometimes I get scared, you know? That you nod your head but just pretend to understand me [uses the 'empty yes' sign]; that you patronize me like other hearing people do."

Now she looked down at the floor. Her tears were poignant remnants of the trauma that she had sustained with hearing persons, beginning with her parents. Her previously unavailable feelings of rage, fear, sadness, and despair now filled the room. Although I had hoped for this moment and had privately predicted it, I nevertheless was slightly shaken.

Ann was also a bit shaken. She appeared both saddened and relieved that our meeting time was up. As much as she had taken two steps forward, she surely felt extremely vulnerable and scared. It was an Ann I had never been allowed to see before. It was an Ann that looked like a child, undoubtedly because a lot of her pain belonged back in her childhood. After we said good-bye, I found myself hoping that she would allow me to see that part of her again.

She cancelled our next appointment, ostensibly because of car trouble. When we met three weeks later, I almost interpreted her missed appointment as a reaction to our last meeting when she had let down her shield. However, I sensed that this would be premature. Now was not the time for me—a hearing psychologist—to prove myself right about her defensive retreat. I simply asked how her car was.

After responding that her car had required a carburetor adjustment, she again resumed her complaining about her boss and other inadequate work accommodations. Although the content was not new, there was a quality of timidity and passivity that I had never seen before. In answer to my question "why don't you stop the interpreter at work when her signs are unclear or demand another one?" she shrugged her shoulders and responded "I can't." She confirmed that she felt helpless and also added that "I've felt this way all my life."

Learned Helplessness

Oppression has varying but profound effects. Many internalize oppression by idealizing hearing people as infallible while devaluing themselves as inferior. Others react in the opposite manner by idealizing themselves and devaluing hearing people. Either way, one is left with a rigid and exaggerated sense of self—too negative or too positive. One therefore cannot flexibly accommodate or adjust to the shifting demands of reality. It becomes difficult to effectively navigate in the world. The oppressed person often ends up feeling overburdened and a sense of pervasive helplessness.

In Ann's case, she often flip-flopped between idealizing her parents as all powerful, knowing figures—"I could never understand what they were saying but it must have been important"—and devaluing them as abusive and "worthless scum." She was left feeling, in her words, like "only half a person." Consequently, although there were currently several bonafide possibilities for her to feel empowered, she adhered to her rigid sense of herself as a helpless victim of circumstance. Those current opportunities seemed too reminiscent of earlier "pseudo-opportunities," which had prompted her to "take the bait" and advocate for herself, only to be thwarted and frustrated. At present, she remained immobilized, bitter, and depressed.

Ann was not alone. Members of any oppressed minority often inherit a legacy that threatens to disempower them— to make them less than they can and ought to be. With reference to the Deaf community in particular, Professor Tom Humphries, who is Deaf, observed "Surrounded by powerful ideas of others that they were less than human, how could deaf mutes conceive of themselves as anything more?"[7]

I wondered aloud to Ann, for the first of what would be many times, what she might be thinking, feeling, or doing with hearing authority figures that gave them more power than they already had. I also bluntly asked Ann how she may be sabotaging herself, for example, by not following her boss's instructions and not showing up for meetings.

This time she did not react with defensive hostility, but instead looked confused. "What do you mean?" she asked.

A good sign, I thought, as it meant the possibility of her accommodating new information. It would be important not to confuse her with too much information or she would reject it as irrelevant or noxious. The delicate balance of therapy. I opted to ask her to revisit a familiar situation in which she had felt disempowered. "Would you tell me again about a painful, oppressive exchange with your parents?" I asked.

"What does that have to do with anything?" she retorted now a bit more defensively.

"A reasonable question," I responded with a smile, "but would you give me some latitude just for a few minutes?" (I felt like Perry Mason asking the judge for some indulgence upon cross examination.)

She nodded her head and gave me the latitude. After hesitating for a few seconds, she recounted a typical family occurrence: "I can remember one time when we were sitting at the dinner table. My brother was excited about something, I think about school. My dad interrupted and looked serious, maybe about money or the car or something. He got angry about what, I don't know. I remember wishing that they wouldn't talk so fast. I then asked my dad what they were talking about but he couldn't understand me. Then my dad said something else to me that was incomprehensible. When I asked him to speak slower, he yelled at me that I should lip-read him better."

"As a hearing person, I can only imagine how that must have felt for you. Pretty awful, huh?"

"You got that right," she answered.

Now that I sensed that we had a more solid collaboration, I could deepen our exploration of how hearing people had come to have so much power. She had just provided the opening we needed. We could now process her experience of speech therapy.

As Ann began recounting her ten years of speech therapy, she dutifully acknowledged her parents' well-meaning intentions to prepare her for the hearing world. Her protection of them, in this regard, was initially puzzling in light of her almost constant vilification of them as "oppressors." I wondered how many times this justification had been drilled into her.

As she continued recalling how horrible speech therapy had been, her stance shifted. Her parents had not viewed speech therapy as a benefit providing Ann with one of many communication options. Instead, they had forbidden her to use any communication means other than speech. They forced her to go, in Ann's words, "to that bastard" three times a week—even while she was at residential school—no matter how much she protested.

In the middle of describing her torment, she abruptly switched from ASL to an English-based visual coding system with fingerspelling, obviously to ensure that what she was about to say was perfectly clear: "My parents were dutifully executing the orders of hearing professionals to exterminate deafness." I got her implication. It had an erie, Nazi-like feel to it.

I decided, somewhat tentatively, to ask Ann to give me more of a feel for—and maybe even to show me—what had happened to her in speech therapy. Her story had to be told. We were in sync as she had anticipated my request. She nodded her head and took a deep breath. Obviously as a necessary preparation, she coiled her body deep into the seat with her eyes looking straight ahead.

As she began to share with me and reexperience her tales of horror, I noticed that her eyes became blank and vacant—similar to what I had witnessed earlier when Ann first described her isolation within her family. Soon her eyes became much more glazed and distant, with a dissociative quality to them, much like one would expect of any post-trauma survivor. She later told me that she had frequent nightmares about her various speech therapists becoming alien monsters gnawing at her, threatening to kill her.

I asked her to describe her thoughts and images, as if they were happening in the present. By this time, she no longer hesitated. At first I could barely make out her words, as she appeared to be vocalizing. Gradually what was happening became clear. Now more loudly and with her eyes closed, she expelled labored, erratic grunting noises that were beyond conscious intention—sounds that sent shivers up my spine.

"G-g-g-g-u, G-g-au, G-g-g-a, Gi, Gish. "G-g-g-g-u, G-g-au, G-g-g-a, Gi, Gish. G-g-g-g-u, G-g-au, G-g-g, Gi, Gish . . ."

She had put herself in a trance state. Her grunts continued for several moments. In the meantime, she had curled into the fetal position in her chair.

I was on the edge of my seat, however. I had not expected this much intensity and what certainly seemed like age-regression. Had we gone too far?

Gradually, her grunts softened and were then replaced by soothing, rocking motions. Ann was also reliving how she undoubtedly had soothed herself as a young child and adolescent. After several more minutes, she opened her eyes and looked up at me.

I nodded. She answered my nod. What had been shared between us could never have been expressed with language. While I had dared to hope for only a "glimpse" of what her speech therapy torture was like, she had permitted me to relive it with her. That night, I, too, had nightmares about alien monsters.

For several sessions, we discussed speech therapy. Now that she felt I understood on a visceral level what it had been like for her (I told her about my nightmares), Ann could openly discuss with me different levels of that experience. She told me how it had been impossible to show her anger directly to her "speech therapist torturers" (even in her dreams) because she had felt so inept and so angry at herself for not achieving oral success. Ann recalled that for many years she became a lifeless robot—a "talking machine." It was a subhuman existence.

Now with her hands clenched in front of her chest, she slowly signed "I want to smack them!" Then she quickly threw down her hands and said "but they smack me instead."

First rage, then despair.

Ann showed up early for her next appointment. Once again, she began by complaining about work: "I was just at a department meeting. People were all talking at once, so fast and the interpreter—who was lousy anyway—couldn't keep up. My boss came in and made some announcement to everyone. Then they laughed about something, but I don't know about what."

Ann's hands were once again clenched, and her face was once again beet red.

It was time to connect her bonafide disempowerment in the past to instances of learned helplessness in the present. "You know, on the one hand, the communication problems at work obviously cause you—as they would almost anybody—to be frustrated and angry, but as you tell the story, it also seems like you're back at the dinner table."

Seeing no protest from Ann, I continued. "You may sometimes react to your boss as if he was your father."

Ann paused for a moment and then slowly nodded her head.

For the remainder of the hour, we worked on exorcising her father from her boss. We talked about the ways she may unconsciously be replicating her past in her present work environment. As she put it, "I need to separate how my boss is really an asshole from how I make him into a bigger one than he really is."

Although she had been reacting to bonafide oppression at work, she had unconsciously exacerbated those noxious conditions by her insubordinate behavior. She then felt as disempowered as she had felt as a child when she was forced into speech therapy. In fact, however, she was more empowered in the present than she was in the past.

Transference

M. Scott Peck defined transference as "an outdated road map."[8] At work, Ann had unconsciously relied on her earlier "map" which showed a world full of debilitating oppression at every corner. By using that "map" to navigate through her present work environment, it became a self-fulfilling prophesy. She helped create what she feared.

I often think back to Ann's stated reason for seeking therapy: to learn how to play politics with hearing people, particularly her boss. She had reportedly chosen me because I was separate from the Deaf community, but I think there was another perhaps more important reason. At some level of awareness, I believe that Ann came to a me as a hearing therapist, not so much because I was separate from her network, but to face and conquer a Goliath figure of sorts.

Whereas she initially viewed me as "unlike those hearing assholes at work," a perception which perhaps I fostered by my initial tacit agreement, she came to view me in accordance with her "map." She soon experienced me as less than ideal, as defective. Ann felt betrayed, perhaps like Dorothy felt when she found that the Wizard of Oz was actually an old man behind the curtain. Eventually, I became the hearing parent, the hearing speech therapist, the hearing boss—the hearing oppressor. I functioned as a psychological "lightning rod"—a catalyst for Ann to unlock her rage and fear with respect to "those hearing others."

I remember initially feeling good, even a bit self-righteous, about my commitment not to oppress Ann like those others. I also remember feeling hurt, even a bit angry, about being defamed by Ann as "one of them." Today, as I reexamine my earlier hurt pride, I have a nagging sense that my commitment to respect others, including Ann, without ever oppressing them is a laudable but elusive goal.

As therapists, we can never be completely free of inadequacy remnants from our inevitably less than perfect childhoods. Feeling damaged ourselves, we may unwittingly become paternalistic over our clients and strive to cure them of those problems that in some way remind us of our own. This is easy to do with Deaf clients. Hearing people are members of a majority who have taken, and have been given, a lot of power to define the lives of Deaf people.

As therapists, it is our ethical responsibility to minimize acts of oppression as much as we are capable. Examining my vulnerabilities in my own psychotherapy has, among other benefits, helped keep my own oppressive impulses in check, but it is a continual, never-ending struggle, a constant accumulation of insight, and a commitment to do it better next time.

Perhaps somehow I did oppress Ann in our sessions, something that I had vowed never to do like those others. Should I have acted as a cross-cultural mediator between Ann and her boss? Did my saying to Ann that I know that hearing people oppress Deaf people put me in the one-up position and deprive her of an important opportunity to teach me that? Was my teaching her about how she may have contributed to her own oppression essentially blaming the victim? These are questions that I still ask.

However, whether I "should have" done this or that, there are important client benefits to having a less-than-perfect therapist. Ann could recover and heal from earlier trauma as we "cocreated" a safe place for us to examine her experiences of oppression not only "out there," but particularly "in here" with me. For the next several sessions, we sorted out those times when she perceived me as acting oppressively and listed how she interpreted my behavior.

1. **True Oppression**

   My using hearing metaphors

   Sometimes being overly preoccupied during our meetings

   Sometimes misunderstanding her

2. **Misinterpreted Oppresion**

   Me feeling smug

Me preferring hearing client

My hoping she gets fired

Sorting out these and other reality-based ("accurate map") and transferentially-based ("outdated map") perceptions was the medicine for her recovery and healing. The process of de-mucking our relationship served as a model for how Ann could demuck her ability to function in the world. Things were going well now. In my notes, I put "rocky road no more."

My error. A few weeks later, Ann stomped into my office and announced that she had gotten a letter of warning, now from the Vice President of the corporation. She requested assistance in composing a letter of response and empha-sized that she wanted no further sessions for a while.

I quickly agreed and helped her compose the letter—to clarify her intent and express her thoughts concisely in Eng-lish. She, however, remained the author; I was simply a coach, a cheering team. For an instant, I asked myself whether I should explore why she wanted to put our visits on hold. I also privately wondered whether my agreeing to her request was appropriate for psychotherapy—maybe it was really education, codependency, or whatever. But no matter how I could have labeled my response to her re-quest, my overriding goal was to empower her.

Two months later, Ann arranged another meeting with me, ostensively to update me on her job situation. We chat-ted about the cast of characters at work, including some "assholes," but unlike before, there were others who were "not so bad." I could not help feeling that I had graduated from the former to the latter category. As we ended our meeting, my hunch was confirmed. Ann warmly shook my hand, made eye contact, and said "I'll see you again when I can. Thank you very much," she smiled.

Again, I was tempted to process with Ann what had changed between us, but now, it seemed more meaningful to nonverbally acknowledge my asshole-no-longer status, our rapproachment. I returned her handshake, smiled, and bid her a warm goodbye.

————

About six months later, Ann sent me a copy of her annual performance review marked "FYI." Her follow-through and attitude at work had significantly improved and she was due for a promotion. However, she wrote in the "employee response" section that the adequacy of accessibility within her work environment had gone from bad to worse. Her letter clearly explained the need for reasonable accommodations, most notably adequately trained interpreters. Her written justification was from the much earlier letter that she had composed with me.

Soon afterward, Ann requested another appointment. She walked into my office appearing quite jubilant. Apparently, shortly after she had given her boss that letter, he gruffly informed her that the company was doing "the best that we can—but don't hold your breath for big changes." However, this time, she explained that rather than "act like an asshole back," she very calmly explained to her boss the criteria of reasonable accommodations and gave him the name of her attorney should he wish further clarification. She thanked him for his time, warmly shook his hand, and wished him a good day.

Two weeks later, her company managed to procure the funds for increased interpreter services, as well as note-takers, visual alarm systems, and a TTY.

Notes

1. Anderson, G.B., & Rosten, E. (1985). In G. B. Anderson & D. Watson, *Counseling deaf people: Research and practice*. Little Rock, AK: Arkansas Rehabilitation Research and Training Center on Deafness and Hearing Impairment.

2. Mindel, E. D., & Vernon, M. (1987). *They grow in silence* (2nd ed.). Boston, MA: Little Brown & Co.

3. Hoffmeister, R. J., & Harvey, M. A. (1996). Is there a psychology of the deaf? In N. S. Glickman & M. A. Harvey (Eds), *Culturally affirmative psychotherapy with deaf persons*. Mahwah, NJ: Lawrence Erlbaum Associates.

4. Vernon, M., & Andrews, J. F. (1990). *The psychology of deafness*. New York: Longman Press.

5. Lane, H. (1992). *The mask of benevolence: Disabling the deaf community*. San Diego. DawnSignPress.

6. Lane, H., Hoffmeister, R., & Bahan, B. (1996). *A journey into the deaf-world*. San Diego, CA: DawnSignPress.

7. Humphries, T. (1996). Of deaf-mutes, the strange, and the modern deaf self. In N.S. Glickman & M. A. Harvey (Eds), *Culturally affirmative psychotherapy with deaf persons*. Mahwah, NJ: Lawrence Erlbaum Associates.

8. Peck, M. S. (1978). *The road less travelled: A new psychology of love, traditional values and spiritual growth*. New York: Simon & Schuster.

CHAPTER NINE

Pockets of Gold

Fifty years after surviving the Bataan Death March and a subsequent forty-two-month internment at a POW slave labor camp, a seventy-year-old veteran was interviewed. He stated that he would not repeat his experiences for a million dollars, but recalled them as the most enriching, ennobling experience of his entire life.[1]

As an adolescent, I would frequently attempt to educate my mother. One afternoon, as we were in the car for an hour, she was captive to a tutorial I called "general insights about life." I ended one segment with an important point I felt she should learn: "there's something good in everything that happens." My mother, usually very calm and accepting, abruptly gave me a sharp, piercing look and quipped "what about your grandfather losing his sight? What's so good about that?" My grandfather was a world-famous cardiologist who had written many books and was trying to write another, but he was going blind. I did not know the answer to her question, but I told her I would think about it. I still do not know the answer and I have been struggling with it for over thirty years.

Thirty-nine-year-old Eric had also struggled with that same question since losing his hearing four years ago. He

144

arrived late for our initial meeting with what seemed like a prepared apology for oversleeping, but it soon became clear that he had been, in his words, "burned by counseling before" and was therefore "iffy" about taking that chance again. However, he was quite depressed.

Soon after becoming deaf, Eric sought counseling from the minister at the Congregational church he attended on a weekly basis. This seemed logical since he led a religious life, but during their first meeting, the minister attempted to comfort Eric with essentially a theological version of my much earlier tutorial to my mother by proclaiming "The Scripture says 'all things work unto good for those who love God.'" Eric, however, was anything but comforted. He recalled the tirade he shot back: "Don't tell me that 'pain builds character'! You think my deafness is good? Has deafness added anything to my character? Oh yes, anger, hostility, frustration, embarrassment, to say nothing of the twenty-four-hour-a-day problems of just trying to get by. Deafness sucks!" Eric then left, slamming the door behind him.

His anger was rekindled at the next church service several days later. He told me about not being able to "take it anymore" and leaving the service, muttering to himself, "Why should I say 'Amen'? An almighty God wouldn't inflict deafness on me like this!" He then headed to the nearest bar. From that moment on, Eric had dismissed God as nonexistent, as dead.

The minister's solace may have been at least partially correct but his timing was certainly way off. From my work with those who have acquired hearing losses, I too have been impressed not only with how many people are able to overcome certain limitations, but also with how some make a leap toward finding psychological and spiritual benefits from the unchangeable.

When I told my mother that I'd think about her question, she politely informed me that I didn't know what I was talking about. Since I didn't have a vision loss myself, what right did I have to suggest that there may be benefits to my grandpa's blindness? I had to admit, at least privately, that she had a valid point.

She still does. I do not have a hearing loss, and so for me to even wonder whether there may be benefits to it might very well be interpreted as arrogance or extreme disrespect. Neither is my intent. Nor would I wish a hearing loss on anyone, including myself, simply to reap possible benefits. I often say that if pain builds character, there surely must be someone else who needs it more than me!

Nevertheless, it seems important to at least speculate about the benefits to hearing loss even though no definitive answers may come forth. I once heard a story about a man who had been looking under a street lamp for several hours for his keys. Finally, a bystander asked him where he had lost them. The man pointed to across the street and replied "over there!"

"But why then," the bystander asked, "are you looking for your keys under the street lamp?"

The man answered confidently, "the light is better over here."

The "light" is certainly better on the topic of coping with hearing loss or going through the grieving process that often goes with it. There is more written about it at least there is the appearance of clarity. While one part of the key to adjustment and coping is, in fact, to learn ways to lessen the negative impact of hearing loss, I continually wonder whether another part of the key is to learn more about its benefits.

I have witnessed many people with acquired hearing losses go through a three-stage process:

1. *The coping stage.* One realizes and begins to actively confront the many subtle yet profound ef-

fects of hearing loss by adopting various coping strategies.

2. *The grieving stage.* One grieves and reluctantly accepts those unchangeable limitations of hearing loss that one cannot change.

3. *The "out of lemons make lemonade" stage.* One experiences a transformation from tolerating what one cannot change to finding ways to benefit from hearing loss.

There are different "levels" of potential benefits. Many anecdotes on the so-called "benefits" of a disability, such as hearing loss, have focussed on what noxious situations one can avoid, i.e., "I'm spared the traffic noise" or "I'll never again have to put up with my husband snoring." A hard-of-hearing man sent me a letter in which he speculated on possible benefits of blindness: "As to being blind, I've thought about the benefits, if any, one could have. We wouldn't see destruction, hatred, and ugliness which occurs everyday." He went on to elucidate one advantage of his own hearing loss: "I don't have to hear my grandchildren argue all of the time."

Acknowledgment of such so-called "benefits" is often very helpful as a rationalization or compensatory strategy, but on a deeper level, these benefits are relatively superficial. After all, there are advantages to hearing traffic noise, at least you know your husband is alive when you hear him snore. And grandchildren arguing can be cute, particularly for grandparents privileged to experience it in short doses.

Other anecdotes of the benefits of hearing loss focus on concrete positive experiences that one can gain instead of on what can be avoided. Some examples are comments such as "I've met some special people that I otherwise wouldn't have met," "I get getting preferential seating," and "the state vocational rehabilitation agency pays for my college."

The following vignette depicts how one woman creatively used her hearing loss to meet interesting people at a party

Paula, a hard-of-hearing woman, asked her hearing friend Betty what she thought of a party. Betty felt awkward about saying that she had enjoyed it. She knew that Paula would certainly have found the party boring and stressful due to her hearing loss.

"It was all right, I guess," Betty meekly replied. "How about you?"

Paula also felt awkward, lest she make Betty feel inadequate about herself. "She doesn't have my gift for meeting people at parties," Paula thought. She looked compassionately at her hearing friend. Every week, Betty would buy various self-help books such as "How to Meet People"; "The One Minute Conversation Opener" and "Nurturing the Inner Shy Child."

Paula smiled silently to herself, as she relived the great party. "Hordes of people are all around me. The noise, the clatter. So I say to that cute guy on my left, 'I'm sorry, I couldn't quite catch what you were saying but it sounded very interesting. I'm hard-of-hearing, you know.'

'Oh, I didn't know that,' he replies with embarrassment.

And I say, 'Could we go to the other room and talk? I really want to understand what you're saying.'

He agrees and wants to know more about my hearing loss. I tell him some typical experiences that hearing people seem to find so fascinating: funny examples of lip-reading faux pas. We laugh. Then he turns his head slightly while saying something to me. Here's my chance to ask him to make eye contact with me, naturally for lip-reading purposes. We laugh some more."

"Enough reminiscing," Paula thought. "How do I answer Betty? How do hearing people cope at parties anyway?"

Paula very tactfully replied "Oh, it was just another party, I guess." (She didn't want to make Betty feel bad.)

Betty was quick to reply in a politically correct, compassionate manner, as she was sensitive to the issues of handicaps. She urged her friend "Don't fret, Paula. Even I found that party boring. I couldn't talk to anyone, you know!" She paused and continued to comfort Paula adding "I know how you must feel."

"Thanks," replied Paula. "It's nice to know that some hearing people actually understand how tough it is to have a hearing loss.

"Poor Betty," Paula thought.

"Poor Paula," Betty thought.

Although there are many other similar gains from hearing loss, these anecdotes still do not get at the more profound "pockets of gold" that one can find, even under what may be layers of grievous pain and distress. Where is, in the words of the Japanese POW quoted at the beginning of this chapter, "the most enriching and ennobling experience"?

Many say such experiences do not exist. In a letter sent to me, one deafened man wrote, "The only good news about hearing loss is an eventual cure." Eric's outburst of "Deafness sucks!" also reflects pain and rage.

A response: Pain, rage, and despair often—although not always—follow traumatic hearing loss. It is indeed important to acknowledge these feelings and not sugar-coat them with positive affirmations. There is an old saying "The barn burned down; now I can see the stars." That's great, but now where do you put the hay? In addition to descriptions of distress from persons with acquired hearing loss, I often hear stories that do not conform to descriptions of relatively superficial advantages, to "coping with disability," or to the "grieving process." Instead, I hear stories of transformation.

Crises have a way of not only crushing but also strengthening the human spirit. Although many clients request psychotherapy only to feel better as they struggle to cope with their hearing loss, there is another challenge—one that is more loosely defined and abstract. It is the challenge of answering the existential and often spiritual questions that their hearing loss has forced on them. In Eric's case, for example, his primary question was "How could God inflict deafness on me?"

Although existential and spiritual questions must be continually asked, they typically have no clear answer. An apparent contradiction to be sure. To respond to these complex questions with neatly packaged answers or affirmations—as Eric's minister did—only addresses these issues in the most superficial way. There are pockets of gold to be found in the eternal struggle to answer unanswerable questions. As psychiatrist Carl Jung stated "When the unstoppable bullet hits the impenetrable wall, we find the religious experience. It is precisely here that one will grow."[2]

Let us struggle to answer the question of what existential and spiritual benefits there are from traumatic hearing loss, knowing full well that the question is fundamentally unanswerable.

Constructing Meaning

Psychiatrist Victor Frankl was a prisoner at Auschwitz during the Holocaust. There he also struggled with how to find benefits from loss, albeit vastly different in scope.

It had been a bad day. We lay in our earthen huts—in a very low mood. Very little was said and every word sounded irritable. Then, to make matters even worse, the lights went out. Tempers reached their lowest ebb. But our senior block warden was a wise man. He improvised a talk about the many comrades who had died in the last few days, either of sickness or of suicide. But he also mentioned what may have been the real reason for their deaths: giving up hope. He maintained that there should be some way of preventing possible future victims from reaching this extreme state. And it was to me that the warden pointed to give this advice.

God knows, I was not in the mood to give psychological explanations or to preach any sermons. I was cold and hungry, irritable and tired, but I had to make the effort and use this unique opportunity. Encouragement was now more necessary than ever.

I spoke of the many opportunities of giving life a meaning. I told my comrades that human life, under any circumstances, never ceases to have a meaning, and that this infinite meaning of life includes suffering. I asked the poor creatures who listened to me attentively in the darkness of the hut to keep their courage in the certainty that the hopelessness of our struggle did not detract from its dignity and its meaning. I said that someone looks down on each of us in difficult hours—a friend, a wife, somebody alive or dead, or a God.

The purpose of my words was to find a full meaning in our life, then and there, in that hut and in that practically hopeless situation. I saw that my efforts had been successful. When the electric bulb flared up again, I saw the miserable figures of my friends limping toward me to thank me with tears in their eyes.[3]

Frankl came to believe that a person's main concern is not to gain pleasure or to avoid pain but rather to find a meaning or purpose in one's life. We do not "search" for meaning in the sense of hoping to find it. Instead, we actively make decisions about what meaning(s) to attribute to certain events, whether to perceive them as good or bad, important or unimportant, half-empty or half-full, opportunity or calamity, etc. Through our internal self-talk, cognitive processes, we create or construct a meaning(s) for an event(s) which then determines how we feel and then what we do.[4]

Unable to end the Holocaust, Frankl actively chose to construct a personal meaning to it; namely, he came to realize that any circumstance—including the Holocaust—can offer a purpose. His particular construction of meaning made him feel more hopeful and contributed to his psychological and spiritual growth through the horrific trauma that he endured. His thoughts and feelings then spurred him to write his seminal book Man's Search for Meaning and to become a renowned psychiatrist.

Hearing loss, while a completely different experience than the Holocaust, may offer an opportunity to create meaning. Again, to quote Carl Jung "One does not become enlightened by imagining figures of light, but by making the darkness conscious."[5] By consciously exploring the "dark" aspects of hearing loss—fear, anger, depression, and anxiety—one can achieve a level of psychological growth that transcends the "acceptance" stage of the grieving process. This odyssey catalyzes a person to construct deeper layers of meanings in their life.

For example, one middle-aged man with acquired deafness wrote me the following note:

Life holds many mysteries that defy answers. Why did so many people have to perish in Oklahoma City? Why did Commerce Secretary Ron Brown and thirty-two others perish in a mission of peace? But we must not use these *unanswerable* [my emphasis] questions as a negative about which to grieve. We can only move forward, positively, doing the best we can in life.

This man explained many world-wide tragedies—in addition to his own—as mysteries for which there are no answers. They had become part of his life that he was obliged to accept. His thoughts—constructions of meaning—enabled him to feel humble and resigned. He then behaved in more purposeful ways, namely, to focus on what he could change—"to move forward."

Many others perceive their hearing loss as giving them a new and worthwhile direction in their lives. Some strive to correct various forms of societal oppression. They become "freedom fighters" against the wrongs of society that have been perpetrated on deaf people. One deafened man, for example, interpreted his loss as offering him a new life's mission. He took it upon himself to scrutinize and help reform the hearing aid industry. The more he experienced frustration and anguish, the more he increased his efforts to improve the lives of other hearing aid users. The more frustration, the more advocacy.

In a very different context, Candice Lyncner founded "Mothers Against Drunk Driving" following the tragic loss of her daughter who was killed by a drunk driver. That tragedy gave renewed purpose to her life.

It was Hillel who asked "If I'm not for myself, who will be for me? If I'm only for myself, what am I?" One's hearing loss may help answer the latter question.

Integrating Duality

An important but difficult lesson about life: To be whole, we have to integrate the myriad dualities which characterize human existence. The following stories will hopefully elucidate this rather abstract concept. One is from a woman who had become deaf while in her late thirties.

> People used to say that everything I touched turned to gold. Everything came easy for me as a child; sports, grades, dates. As an adult, I graduated college, fell into a job as an editor, and lived a fantasy kind of existence. But then I lost some of my hearing and soon I became deaf. For the first time, life became difficult. There were many things I couldn't do no matter how much I tried. Painful as it was (and still is) I can honestly tell you that I have grown more in the last year than in the first thirty-five years of my life. I now appreciate what I have; I take the time to acknowledge how hard I have worked to be included at work and I like myself more. Sort of funny isn't it, how it happened?

The addition of difficulty to her life helped her cherish the easy parts more and reexamine what was truly important. That easy–difficult duality added more contrast and texture to her experience of herself and her world.

Oncologist Bernie Siegel wrote about many of his patients who were confronted with an existential duality; those who, in his words, "have sort of died to stay alive." He explains

> I'm talking about your becoming who you didn't want to be, because of pressure from parents or other authority figures—you become the doctor, the teacher, the plumber, the housewife, even if the work and role are meaningless to you. And then one day you are told you have a year to live. For some of you, learning that you are mortal finally gives you permission to live your life.[6]

Finally, there is Goethe's King Faust story, written almost 200 years ago in 1808. Faust, who was revered by everyone in his kingdom, was celebrating his good fortune with all of his subjects. It was a perfect day with perfect music, libation, ornate decor, and so on, but at the height of all the pomp and circumstance, a smelly, wet, dirty dog ran in and promptly jumped on the King, threatening to ruin the event. However, the King did not attempt to rid himself of this burden, but embraced it! He realized that he needed to come to terms with—to integrate—his dark, disowned side, symbolized by the dog, before he could attain true wisdom and happiness. Faust needed to examine and integrate his pain to feel whole and fulfilled. Again, an essential duality.

We are all affected by myriad dualities—the Yin and the Yang. Typically, we welcome one pole of the duality while we fail to acknowledge or reject the other pole: what Carl Jung called "the shadow." This is the disowned part of us that is the repository for those memories, thoughts, and feelings that cause us distress. Nevertheless, as the previous stories illustrate, there are important psychological benefits to integrating one's shadow.

By integrating our shadow, we find the pockets of gold that are contained within it. This odyssey gives perspective and energy to our lives. As poet William Blake put it "we should go to heaven for form and to hell for energy- and marry the two. When we can face our inner heaven and our inner hell, this is the highest form of creativity."[7] Indeed, it may be that the tension within this duality is what fuels creativity. Psychoanalyst Alice Miller, for example, has speculated about the positive influences of early trauma on the creative works of Pablo Picasso, Buster Keaton, and Friedrich Nietzsche.[8]

Integrating our shadow does not mean succumbing to it. Bernie Siegel, for example, would never recommend that his patients resign themselves to cancer. We do not have to choose between ignoring the pains of loss and being completely consumed by it. We can learn to place the pain of loss slightly off to the side of our visual field, where we can keep an eye on it while enjoying other sites, instead of in the center of our visual field, where it would forever cast a pervasively ominous cloud.

Somehow sweet nectar tastes even sweeter when we remind ourselves that the supply is limited.

Heaven and hell, happiness and misery exist by virtue of their contrast to the other. They are dialectics. As a popular example, where would Luke Skywalker be without Darth Vader?

Connection and Compassion

It was Elie Wiesel who observed that the "human condition [is] to be alone but faced with another person being alone. If you face someone, your child or your wife or your friend, then you can find out who you are, but the other one is essential, indispensable."[9] We need to connect with and have compassion for "the other one" to realize our human potential.

Who is "the other one?" There are two levels of human connections: with the particular and with the universal. For our present discussion, the particular level is when one identifies and connects with other people who have acquired hearing losses; "only another person like me can understand my unique joys and anguishes." Indeed this is one function of peer organizations such as the National Association of the Deaf, Self Help for the Hard-of-Hearing, and the Association of Late-Deafened Adults. Particular level connections are both precious and essential. However, in my opinion, they are incomplete.

The universal level does not emphasize one's uniqueness but that "we are all human." It helps us connect with the joys and anguish of humanity. As an illustration, there is a story from the time of the Buddha. Kisa, a young woman, married a man who loved her very much. In time, she gave birth to a son. She and her husband were exquisitely joyful and lived together quite happily. Sadly, two years after their son was born, the child became ill and died very quickly. Kisa was devastated; her heart was broken. She was so stricken with grief that she refused to admit that her son had died. She carried his small corpse around, asking everyone she met for medicine to make her boy well again.

Kisa went to the Buddha and asked him if he could please cure her son. The Buddha looked at Kisa with deep love. He said, "Yes, I will help you, but first I need a handful of mustard seed." When Kisa in her joy promised to collect the seed immediately, the Buddha added, "but the mustard seed must be taken from a house in which no one has lost a child, husband, wife, parent, or friend. Each seed must come from a house that has not known death."

Kisa went from house to house asking for the mustard seed, and always the response was the same: "Yes, we will gladly give you some mustard seed, but alas, the living are few and the dead are many." Each had lost a father or mother, husband or wife, son or daughter. She visited one home after another, and every home told the same story. By the time she got to the end of the village, her eyes were opened, and she saw the universality of sorrow. Everyone had experienced some great loss; each had felt tremendous grief. Kisa realized that she was not alone in her suffering; her sorrow had given birth to a compassion for the larger human family. Thus, Kisa was finally able to grieve the death of her son and bury him, and she returned to the Buddha to thank him and receive his teachings.

The universal level is also valid but incomplete. Loss and sorrow are universal, but each person's particular suffering is nevertheless unique. The feelings that come with acquired hearing loss are both different and the same as what comes with other losses. Another duality.

Eric

No benefits of hearing loss seemed relevant to Eric when I met first him. He judged his life as having "enough" meaning prior to his hearing loss. He had easily accepted the duality of the ups and the downs, and he had enjoyed hanging out with people both similar and dissimilar to himself. Eric wanted none of that "silver lining bullshit" that he had gotten from his minister and I was not about to give it to him.

Our task was to address and change how his life was falling apart. He had emotionally withdrawn from his wife and family. His work performance as a mail carrier was slipping. Socially, he used to hang out with his buddies, usually to shoot darts, his favorite hobby. He had even won several state competitions before becoming deaf, but that was all in the past. His life was now melancholy. He spent his time at home by himself, often in front of the TV, with beer in hand.

For the next several months we discussed the various psychological effects of his hearing loss as well as what coping strategies he could use. He also allowed himself to grieve about what he could not change. Gradually he became less depressed.

One day he appeared at my door and proudly announced that he just won a local dart competition after practicing for "only a day!" His relationships had also improved. For example, he was looking forward to spending Father's Day with his family. Maybe he would invite some friends to join the party! Work was also going better. Eric was clearly "getting back to his old self."

At the beginning of one meeting, I asked him what else he would like to work on. "After all," I said, "you've made your life go much better."

He thought for a moment and agreed that he indeed was much less depressed. Then, after thinking some more, he added "I still feel that something's missing, a kind of emptiness, a void that I don't remember feeling before I became deaf."

"You mean since you slammed the door on God?" I asked.

Although my question seemed to come from left field, it felt quite relevant. It was a question that would have once been uncharacteristic of me to ask. Without missing a beat, Eric nodded his head. Prior to his hearing loss, his spiritual beliefs—the foundation of his life—did not account for undeserved suffering. Bad things could not happen to good people. He did not find solace in biblical stories, such as the story of Job, which would have justified and even deified his suffering. Instead, Eric deemed God as having committed the ultimate sin against him. When Eric slamming the door on his minister, he had slammed the door on God. He had sentenced God to death.

Eric was not alone with his spiritual outrage. Such befuddled betrayal is a common experience for a religious or spiritual person who has learned about and/or personally experienced any kind of traumatic loss. Throughout our history, humankind has wrestled with whether to hold God accountable for what has gone wrong in a world which presumably has been under divine control.

Like many others, Eric was left with what author Karen Armstrong called our culture's "God-hole": our rejection and abandonment of God, leaving one with a spiritual void, an emptiness, a deadness.[10] While negating God provided Eric with clear answers to all the "why" questions, it left a hole that could not be filled by family rituals or by winning dart competitions.

The deadness and void that remained was not due to depression. As Eric so poignantly put it, "I realize that by killing God, I had killed part of myself." He felt cut off not only from the church community, but also from a divine presence, one that had helped him to never feel alone. He remained a spiritual amputee.

"Maybe your deafness has prepared you for a different level of discussion with God?" I offered.

Eric was one step ahead of me. He had already telephoned his minister to make an appointment. He was now ready to continue the conversation that was interrupted five years ago. As it turned out, his minister had been hoping for this opportunity, lamenting his much earlier "error in timing." There would be no more simple answers to complex questions.

Several weeks later, Eric gave me a vivid account of their meeting. The minister offered no platitudes. Instead, he invited Eric to wrestle with God, much like many others had done before him. He was invited to vent his rage at God and demand an explanation. When he could find none, the minister offered only his sincere empathy and condolences. "If only there were clear answers," the minister would repeatedly say. In this manner, he validated Eric's loss of an omnipotent, omniscient, benevolent God that would always make sure that nothing bad would happen. That God had died.

Eric was helped not simply to recapture what he had lost—to return to his predeafness level of spiritual development—but also to evolve in his spirituality. He continued a long tradition throughout humankind of coming to terms with so-called "unfair" acts in the world. Now his evolving conception of God had to account for the duality of fair and unfair. Soon he resumed attending Church services regularly, but experienced the teachings much differently than he had before.

As Eric learned to tolerate and then appreciate the dualities inherent in his God, he also learned the same lessons with respect to himself. They were parallel processes; his God had a shadow and so did he. Like King Faust, Eric allowed himself to fully experience and "embrace" his shadow. His "shadow" contained his distress from his deafness as well as other "smelly, wet, dirty dogs." He not only grieved and learned to manage his shadow, but also used it to find those deeper levels of life's richness and texture that one only experiences while simultaneously holding life's agony and ecstasy in his soul.

For example, in his own words, "My wife thought that I had gone off my rocker the other day at the Art museum. It was something I could not explain at first. I usually don't cry, certainly not from simply looking at a painting. But there I was—staring at a beautiful landscape with vivid oranges, reds, and blue sky. I burst into tears! Before, when my life wasn't so bloody difficult, I would never have appreciated such a beautiful painting!"

His life now had deeper levels of meaning. The quality of his connections with others also changed. He proudly reported that he had joined town meetings to advocate for disabled persons' rights. His interest in dart competitions continued—in fact, he won more tournaments—but his social activities broadened to include "more intimate discussions with friends."

There is a Buddhist saying that when the student is ready, the teacher will come. Eric's hearing loss had become his teacher.

———

As Eric was leaving my office one day, he remarked, "Ya know Mike, I was a hell of a lot happier thinking that life was fair before I became deaf, but I'm a lot wiser now."

His off-handed remark echoed a profound truth that every human experience can be expressed in terms of a paradox. In this case, less happy but more wise. Triumph and recovery do not mean living happily ever after. Nor do they mean a guarantee of no more suffering. Instead, "finding the pockets of gold" can be a way to come to terms with this profound duality, to integrate it and hold it dearly in one's consciousness.

Before Eric left, I instinctively asked him, "If you could, would you trade wisdom for happiness?"

His answer was quick and to the point: "To be honest with you—yeah, sure I would, but I can't go backwards in time. So I'll have to take wisdom."

Like the veteran from the POW camp, Eric would not have wished his own traumatic hearing loss for "a million dollars," but it had become the most enriching, ennobling experience of his entire life.

Notes

1. Sipprelle (1992). In Meichenbaum, D. (1994). *A clinical handbook/practical therapist manual: For assessing and treating adults with post-traumatic stress disorder (PTSD)*. Waterloo, Ontario, Canada: Institute Press.

2. Johnson, R., (1991). *Owning your own shadow*. San Fransisco, CA: Harper & Row.

3. Frankl, V. E. (1963). *Man's search for meaning*. New York: Pocket Books.

4. Meichenbaum, D. (1977). *Cognitive-behavior modification: An integrative approach*. New York: Plenum Publishing.

5. Johnson, *Owning your own shadow.*

6. Siegel, B. (1990). *Love medicine and miracles*. New York: Harper Collins.

7. Johnson, *Owning your own shadow.*

8. Miller, A. (1990). *The untouched key: Tracing childhood trauma in creativity and destructiveness*. New York: Doubleday.

9. Brown, R. M. (1989). *Elie Wiesel: Messenger to all humanity—revised edition*. Notre Dame, IN: University of Notre Dame Press.

10. Armstrong, K. (1993). *A history of God*. New York: Ballantine Books.

CHAPTER TEN

The Anatomy of Trauma and Triumph

I'm here at the suggestion of Dr. Smith," offered Donna. "It's very nice to meet you," I replied. "How does Dr. Smith think I can help?"

Standard opening introductions. I imagined the subtext of Donna's statement to be that although she came of her own free will, she did not quite know for what purpose, other than perhaps to mollify her doctor. Perhaps she felt more comfortable starting with safe conversational topics before more personal matters. I affirmed and welcomed her decision to come and added an indirect question, the subtext of which was "aside from Dr. Smith, how do you think I can help?"

When I met Donna, she was twenty-seven years old and had a progressive hearing loss, cause unknown. Despite this, however, she seemed completely composed and in control of her life. She had repeatedly told her doctor that she was strong, confident in her abilities, and could overcome all obstacles associated with hearing loss: "It's really quite simple: I refuse to let it run my life!" she routinely proclaimed. She used the top-of-the-line hearing aids, had convinced her company to purchase a variety of assistive listening devices, and knew the ADA (American Disabilities Act) practically by heart. Donna did not want her doctor's sympathy nor did she want mine.

When her physician made the referral to me, he emphasized his genuine respect for her survival skills and tenacity, adding that "I wish my other patients would learn some of her coping skills." However, to his credit, he did not take her self-affirming statements at face value but rather looked beneath the surface and acknowledged their complexity. He wondered whether her confidant and composed presentation—although genuine—was incomplete; whether, alongside her composure, she was also experiencing private *dis*composure and fear.

I asked Donna to take a guess about what Dr. Smith's concerns were. As she pondered the question, her composure crumbled a bit. She quickly recovered, and then slowly and carefully proceeded—in her words—to "take a guess."

"Dr. Smith probably told you how helpless and defeated I feel; like the rug keeps getting pulled out from under me or something like that."

She could not have said it more succinctly. I complemented Donna on her perceptiveness and privately noted the obvious—that her conjecture reflected not only her intuition and alliance with Dr. Smith, but also her projection of her own anxieties onto him. At this young stage of our relationship, it was undoubtedly safer for Donna to let Dr. Smith become the voice for her own fears and anxieties.

As Donna and I ended our first meeting, I confirmed that Dr. Smith and I had, in fact, agreed on "something like that," namely, how psychologically traumatic hearing loss could be.

A Theoretical Look at Trauma

A common definition of trauma from the mental health literature is an event that: (1) falls outside the range of ordinary human experience, (2) exceeds the individual's per-ceived coping abilities, and (3) significantly disrupts that individual's psychological functioning.[1]

Acquired deafness clearly falls outside the range of or-dinary human experience in that it does not happen to most people. However, the onset of deafness may or may not exceed a particular individual's coping abilities and may or may not significantly disrupt an individual's psychologi-cal functioning. Stated differently, a loss is traumatic to the degree that it disrupts the psychological integrity of an in-dividual. A collapse of psychological integrity is one com-mon thread among the many descriptions of trauma, that it causes "a tearing apart of self-protection,"[2] "a breakdown of one's basic theory of reality,"[3] and a "shattering or fragmen-tation of self."[4, 5]

This description by itself, however, is inadequate. In my first meeting with Donna, for example, she indeed ap-peared composed—as having psychological integrity—but was she really? What does psychological integrity look like? How do we describe it? How do we know whether one's hearing loss results in a collapse of psychological integrity?

The different building blocks of integrity have to do with our fundamental psychological needs.6 We share many—if not all—of the following needs, albeit with much variation in inclusion and emphasis:*

> **Frame of reference**—The need to view the world as just, meaningful, stable, and controllable.
>
> **Safety**—The need to feel reasonably secure from harm.
>
> **Intimacy/trust**—The need to feel connected to and validated by others; to believe in the word of another.

---

*This list is an adaptation of McCann and Pearlman's model in accor-dance with my clinical experience.

Independence—The need to feel empowered; to control one's own life.

Cultural affiliation—The need to belong to a larger community or cultural group.

Esteem—The need for self approval; to be valued by oneself.

Power—The need to exert control over others.

Existential meaning—The need for purpose in one's life.

Spirituality—The need to feel connected to a higher power which transcends secular experience.

As part of an Association of Late-Deafened Adults (A.L.D.A.) national conference, I asked participants to describe how their own hearing losses had affected the fulfillment of these different need areas. The following responses are representative of the audience, all of whom had experienced hearing losses during their late adolescence or adulthood.

Frame of reference: "My hearing loss . . .

— made my world full of randomness.

— destroyed what might have been.

— made me see that bad things happen to good people.

— threw me off balance.

— changed my world."

Safety: "My hearing loss . . .

— meant danger—not hearing someone coming

— made me worry what if someone is breaking in? Theft? Fire? Being attacked from behind?

— made me fear ridicule and discrimination.

— terrifies me, makes me feel claustrophobic."

Intimacy/trust: "My hearing loss . . .

— builds walls between me and my family.

— makes me tempted to reject others before they reject me.

— creates a crisis for me of what to do after saying hello.

— thwarts my spontaneity with romance.

— feels like a glass wall.

— leads other people to minimize it, to tell me to 'try harder.'

— . . . I've come to find out who my friends really are."

Independence: "My hearing loss . . .

— has forced me to redefine independence–dependence issues as not all or nothings.

— lowers my financial earning power.

— has taught me to cherish aloneness.

— is surmountable. I don't need help to get over it.

— . . . I feel empowered.

— . . . I feel too dependent."

Cultural affiliation: "My hearing loss . . .

— has created an identity crisis.

— . . . I don't know sign language but I'm deaf.

— . . . The Deaf community rejects me. The hearing community rejects me. Where am I?

— . . . I'm neither in the hearing or Deaf culture; I'm in A.L.D.A."

Esteem: "My hearing loss . . .

— feels demeaning.

— . . . I have sudden feelings of embarrassment and feeling stupid.

— . . . My self concept goes up and down.

— . . . I feel compelled to show my competence.

— . . . I must control how much of my sense of self is polluted by hearing loss.

— . . . I feel inadequate, without self respect."

Power: "My hearing loss . . .

— has forced me to learn and practice self advocacy.

— tempts to me do violence.

— makes me aware of my ability to control my world. I need to figure out how.

— . . . The Serenity prayer. I don't have to control everything but I can control a great deal.

— . . . I have the power to decide who to educate; I can't educate everybody."

Existential meaning: "My hearing loss . . .

— ended my former life and made my new life begin.

— has helped me integrate the light and dark dualities of my life.

— puts me in touch with my death.

— has taught me what's important in my life.

— gives purpose to my life.

— has expanded my experience of humanness."

Spirituality: "My hearing loss . . .

— has begun a spiritual quest for me.

— makes me stronger spiritually.

— teaches me that humility is okay, and that there's a higher power.

— has changed my spiritual path.

— . . . appreciate group church less; I pray more individually."

With this framework, we can now begin to understand the complexity of how hearing loss may affect a particular individual. A brief review: I began by stating that acquired hearing loss is traumatic to the extent that it disrupts the psychological integrity of an individual. I then analyzed the components of that integrity as comprising the fulfillment of different needs.

We now take our analysis a step further with a hypothetical situation, admittedly oversimplified. Suppose two people sustain a hearing loss: a "people-oriented person," who cherishes conversation and a "thing-oriented person," who cherishes mostly machines and technology. In as much as deafness primarily creates a conversational barrier with respect to the hearing world (recall Helen Keller's axiom that blindness separates you from things, deafness separates you from people) then we would predict that the people-oriented person would be more traumatized by acquired deafness.

People have a varying hierarchy of needs—that is, particular needs which are more central to maintaining their equilibrium or "integrity" as contrasted with other needs which remain more peripheral. If an event disrupts the satisfaction of central needs, then trauma results; if an event threatens only peripheral needs, then a lesser reaction would be predicted. In this regard, whether or not the event itself happens infrequently is a relatively unimportant factor influencing how that event is experienced. Commonplace events can be experienced as traumatic.

Take a trivial example. Hardly a week goes by when someone does not cut in front of me in line. I may hardly take notice of this ordinary act—although I perceive it to be unfair—because I have learned not to depend on the world as a fair place. However, if, in order for me to feel intact, I must absolutely view each and every minute event in the world as fair and predictable—if a stable frame of reference is central to my system of needs or to my basic integrity—then I will be significantly more bothered by that unfair event. In fact, I may experience trauma—a significant disruption of psychological integrity—from that commonplace, seemingly nontraumatic event.

There are five factors that influence the experience of trauma, in this case, catalyzed by the person cutting in line:

1. *The event*

   A person cuts in line.

2. *The objective effects of the event*

   I will wait longer in line and arrive home late for dinner.

3. *One's perception of the event*

   It exemplifies oppression, unfairness.

4. *The psychological effects of one's perception on need satisfaction*

   It threatens my frame of reference needs.

5. *How central or peripheral those affected psychological needs are*

   A completely fair and just world is essential to me.

In this case, my experience of trauma from the person cutting in line was that the event disrupted a central frame of reference need. It was not due to objective effects of the event.

Let us return to the event of acquired hearing loss. Its so-called objective effects have been illustrated in other chapters, i.e., the chapter titled "Changing the Rules of Trivial Pursuit," but that is not the full story. Donna as well as many others in this book exemplifies that the potentially traumatic effects of hearing loss depend on how one perceives it, specifically on what central needs are affected.

As we noticed from the A.L.D.A. conference proceedings, some people perceive their hearing loss as signaling danger, as thwarting the fulfillment of their safety needs, i.e., "not hearing someone coming." If safety needs are central to a person's sense of integrity, then that person will experience hearing loss as traumatic. If, however, that particular person deems, let's say, spiritual needs to be central and safety to be of far lesser importance, than that individual is likely to experience his/her hearing loss as only stressful, but not as traumatic per se.

Donna

One day I asked Donna to tell me more about Dr. Smith's views on "how helpless and defeated you feel; like the rug keeps getting pulled out from under you or something like that."

She smiled, understanding my reference to what she had said during our initial visit. "I guess you knew back then that I was talking about me, huh?"

"I had a 50–50 chance of being right, didn't I?" We laughed and Donna nodded her head. "Would you tell me more about the rug?" I asked.

"Ever since I was a kid," she began, "I've had to be basically self-sufficient, depending on myself, for example, to pack my lunches for school, to make sure I knew the bus schedule, and to do the laundry and the food shopping. As soon as I could, I got a part-time job at a supermarket so I could buy my own clothes and other things for the house. You see, my parents were divorced when I was seven years old and my dad skipped town without paying child support. My mom worked two or three jobs and wasn't home most of the time. I was the one who took care of my two younger brothers. They depended on me for a lot. Although I resented it sometimes, the bottom line was I felt proud of what I did."

"You should have felt proud. You did a lot! So is your 'rug' your self-sufficiency, independence? Being the one others depend on?"

"Definitely! I've learned to depend on me, myself and I," she emphasized. "I trust myself more than I trust anyone else. My independence means a lot to me!"

"So has your hearing loss affected your sense of your own independence?" I asked.

"How could it not!" she exclaimed. Whereas her countenance had been calm and self-assured, it was as though a switch had suddenly been activated, rendering her fearful, angry, and vulnerable.

"My earning power is much lower. Suddenly I have to beg people to talk clearly and repeat themselves. Half the time I can't even understand those damn answering machines (they're set at the wrong frequency). Peoples' voices sound garbled on the phone. Using a TTY isn't fast enough and. . . ."

Donna generated a long list of how she perceived her hearing loss as primarily thwarting the fulfillment of her independence needs. She showed me quite vividly what, as Dr. Smith had conjectured, lied underneath her presentation of composure and self-confidence. As Donna clutched the arms of her chair, I imagined her clutching a ledge on a tall building for fear that she would fall off.

Her independence had been most important and central in defining her identity and ensuring her stable functioning. The rug getting pulled away from her was her metaphor for collapsed integrity—psychological fragmentation of self. That was what had made her hearing loss so traumatic. I wondered, however, whether her independence stood alone or whether it was part of a constellation of central needs.

"As a child, you became not only independent as a way of separating from your family, but also a surrogate parent of sorts, hmm?" I asked.

"Yeah, someone had to do it. My mother couldn't do it!"

"How did you feel taking on that role?"

"A mixture of feelings: anger, fear of all the responsibility, pride. Most of all, it felt like the right thing to do. It felt good!"

"And do you help and nurture others now and feel good about it?" I asked.

She laughed and squirmed uncomfortably in her seat. I sensed that I had touched a nerve, but wasn't sure exactly which one.

"Now people help and try to nurture me! Before it meant a lot to me to help others. It gave my life meaning."

This time I laughed privately to myself. It was as if Donna had memorized the need entitled Existential meaning: The need for purpose in one's life. Being a surrogate parent as a child—and, as an adult, helping others—gave her life a sense of purpose. Feeling like she had lost that because of her hearing loss was another part of her "rug."

Donna suddenly looked much younger and fearful: her eye contact with me became scattered, she became fidgety in her seat, and she began to laugh nervously. I thought I noticed a slight trembling of her legs. My guess was that fear was one emotion she had not allowed herself to feel as a child, as she was burdened by too many other responsibilities.

I was tempted to travel back in time to her childhood and to help her amplify her feelings—perhaps to see what anger may be looming under her fears and responsibilities—but now it felt more productive to help her compensate for her inevitable feelings of reduced independence and existential meaning by helping her fulfill other needs that perhaps had been relatively dormant until now. I wanted to tap into some of her obvious strengths.

Rebalancing Donna's System of Needs

I asked Donna to visualize her nine needs (outlined earlier) as nine individual people standing in a circle facing each other. I then asked her to consider what Independence might say to Power?"

At first she smirked and then furrowed her eyebrows while waving her hands to dismiss the question. I persisted and asked her to wonder aloud with me. "Tell me, Dr. Harvey, when did you begin to see all these little people?" she asked.

We laughed. Seeing no protest from her—and even some humor in its place—I took the lead and began staging a long, imaginary psychodrama. "Maybe Independence might complain to Power that 'I hate how dependent I feel!'"

"Yeah, yeah, that's how I feel, so dependent!" Donna interrupted.

I acknowledged her reaction and continued: "So then Independence might ask Power for some help. 'Hey, Power! What do I do with these yucky feelings of dependence? I hate them!'

"Power might assure her that 'you don't necessarily lose power by depending on others; you can actually come to feel more empowered by allowing yourself to depend on others, as opposed to remaining autonomous and isolated.' Power may then share the teachings of the women's movement which has helped both women and men acknowledge that too much autonomy and independence is suffocating."[7]

Donna was obviously enjoying the play and appeared to relate to the imaginary dialogues between the "parts" of herself. I, too, was enjoying myself.

"Now Intimacy/trust and Cultural affiliation chime in: 'You're right! Independence can be very lonely and limiting. We grow through our intimate connections with others and through our cultural heritage. Donna should join some peer organizations, expand her social network, and meet other people who have acquired hearing losses. She should take advantage of this tremendous growth opportunity. Let's find out what Esteem has to say on this matter.'

"Esteem responds: 'All of this is fine and good, but she needs to feel that she deserves growth and intimacy—that she's a good enough person. I can help her with that.'

"The remaining needs all acknowledge Esteem's role and give their thanks. Now they are curious about what Frame of reference and Existential meaning have to offer. They now respond: 'Whereas we once thought that our world is fair and just—each independent person for herself—we have learned that it is not. After an initial shock, we have come to understand that connecting with others in a meaningful way can also give Donna a purpose to her life.'

"The Safety need overhears this conversation and can't help adding, 'don't forget that there's also safety in numbers. Man and Woman weren't designed to be alone.'

"The other needs thank her in unison. (I was getting into playing the different roles, a frustrated actor perhaps.)

"Spirituality elaborates about the 'oneness of the world—and that everybody and everything in the world is a manifestation of that oneness (Genesis 1:27). Donna is always with God. Even God needs reasonable accommodations.'

"The group caucuses. Independence protests as she feels ganged up on: 'There's nothing so terrible about independence, you know.'

"'There's nothing so great about it either, you know,' the group retorts.

"'I don't like the way you're talking to me,' Independence counters.

"Now an argument ensues, some infantile name calling, the pace quickens, all of the needs are speaking at the same time, it's getting out of hand. Donna, what do we do?"

I continued to plead with Donna who, by this time, was clapping.

She finally answered my plea: "Now all you nine girls—stop fighting or you'll all go to your rooms. [laughter] There's room for all of you. Dr. Harvey, that means you, too." [more laughter]

In fact, there was "room" for Donna's needs not only to coexist but also to nurture each other. In other words, she could reprioritize and rebalance her system of needs. Given the assault on her sense of independence, the task was to make that need less central—to contain the wound to her sense of independence—and to increase the importance and successful fulfillment of her remaining needs.

With our imaginary psychodrama as a backdrop to our continued discussions, Donna began fostering more intimate relationships than she had time to develop before her hearing loss. Real dialogue assumed central importance, whereas her prior pseudo-independence—"the I don't need anyone but me attitude"—had once consumed her energies. She commented quite frequently that having to directly focus on others and make eye contact—essential for lip-reading—helped foster intimate and meaningful exchange. As Donna put it, "it created an island with another in the midst of chaos."

Donna also began to attend synagogue services. She could not follow most of the service, even though an FM system had been installed, but this felt okay as each snippet of ideas that she caught served as a starting point for her own internal dialogue, meditation, and ultimately her experience of the divine. Moreover, in her words, she had never been "a group person" anyway. She observed "Aren't religious experiences essentially private?" In this manner, her sense of independence now reemerged in the context of fulfilling her spiritual needs.

––––

One day Donna mentioned that she had seen Dr. Smith for a routine medical checkup. As he had originally referred her for psychotherapy, he was curious about how our sessions had been going. I asked Donna if she thought her doctor still regarded her as feeling "helpless" and "defeated."

She admitted that "the rug still keeps getting pulled from under me" but added that "somehow I don't feel so helpless and defeated anymore." As she contemplated that paradox, she observed "my life doesn't seem so simple anymore."

Donna and I had worked together for a little under 1 year. Several years after we had parted, she sent me a Peanuts cartoon with the caption "the secret of life is to look good at a distance."

Underneath the script, she wrote:

Dear Mike,

Like Peanuts, I, too, have learned that we look good only at distance. It's not that we necessarily look all bad at close range. Rather, the more I understand myself, the more I come to appreciate how complex things really are. What was once black and white is now a mosaic, and for that I am glad.

That's now the secret of my life.

When I become overwhelmed with life's complexity and wish things were clear and uncomplicated, I often think of Donna's life becoming a "mosaic." I, too, would ultimately rather have it that way.

Notes

1. McCann, L. & Pearlman, L. A. (1990). *Psychological trauma and the adult survivor: Theory, therapy, and transformation.* New York: Brunner/Mazel.

2. Herman, J. L. (1992). *Trauma and recovery.* New York: Basic books.

3. Epstein, S. (1991). The self-concept, the traumatic neurosis, and the structure of personality. In D. Ozer; J. M. Healy, Jr. & A. J. Steward (Eds.), *Perspectives on personality* (Vol. 3). London: Jessica Kingsley.

4. Ulman, R., and Brothers, D. (1988). *The shattered self: A psychoanalytic study of trauma.* Hillsdale, N.J.: Analytic Press.

5. Kohut, H. (1971). *The analysis of the self.* New York: International University Press.

6. McCann, *Psychological trauma.*

7. Jordan, J. V., Kaplan, A. G., Miller, J. B., & Stiver, I. (1991). *Woman's growth through connection: Writings from the Stone Center.* New York: Guilford.

CHAPTER ELEVEN

Resilience to Trauma: An Inspirational Voice from Cyberspace

Carol was the first to raise her hand after I finished my speech at an out of state convention. "Dr. Harvey, how exactly does one triumph over hearing loss?"

I looked at my watch and was relieved that there were only two minutes left. After I don't remember how many "ums," I managed to recall what a mentor had once told me when I asked him that very same question about trauma: "In order to triumph over trauma," he said, "one should seek to better understand it and then share those insights with supportive others." I imparted those words of wisdom to Carol and time was up, but I invited her to e-mail me for further conversation.

We have been corresponding via e-mail ever since that speech five years ago, back in the days of the 286 Intel chip.

In her first e-mail message, Carol introduced herself as one who leads a successful, fulfilling, and challenging life. "I have a wonderful family which includes my husband of almost twenty-five years and two teenage children," she began. "Professionally, I have a doctorate in Sociology and am on the faculty at an Ivy League University. My career keeps me quite busy and stimulated. I feel very fortunate."

I imagined her sitting in an impressively cluttered university office with shelves of books, reams of research proposals, graduate students running in and out, and a computer, and then driving home to her family, a beautiful house with a two-car garage, a big yard, and perhaps a dog or a cat. However, the description of her obvious success and happiness was in stark contrast to the next paragraph in which she described how she had lost her hearing:

> About thirty years ago, when I had just turned twenty-one, I was driving around with a bunch of friends on a beautiful summer day. We were stopped at an intersection when a drunk driver hit us head-on. The next thing I knew, I woke up in a hospital, having been in a coma for several days. I found out later that all my friends in the car had been killed instantly. I very clearly remember, as if it were yesterday, lying there watching peoples' mouths move but being unable to hear their words. My hearing was completely gone!

> For several long months, I lay in traction, hooked up to a bunch of machines with many tubes coming out of my body—trapped in a suddenly silent world that I didn't understand. To say that losing all my hearing was traumatic is a gross understatement, but I eventually got back on my feet again. My dad always used to say, "you gotta get up a third time after they've pushed you down twice."

She ended her e-mail simply with "Looking forward to hearing from you."

Carol's introductory e-mail contained what had become a familiar duality of peoples' lives: their joys and achievements juxtaposed with their sorrows and losses. Both are primal stories. Success stories are easy to share, perhaps even easy to boast about. The other stories involving themes of pain, however, are more intimate, precisely because they are more difficult to share. As such, their disclosure often signals the beginning of a true friendship.

I postponed responding to her e-mail until the next day, as it was late. I was also in the middle of reading a book by one of my favorite authors, Ernest Hemingway, and was impatient to return to it. As I was about to put down *A Farewell to Arms* for the night, two sentences immediately jumped out at me: "The world breaks everyone. And afterward some are strong in the broken places."1 I thought of Carol and then fell asleep.

Between appointments the next afternoon I recalled her letter in which she articulately described how the world had "broken" her, but what was most striking was her apparent resiliency, her getting back on her feet, in her father's words, "a third time" and achieving impressive personal and professional successes. At least from what I was able to glean from her initial correspondence, somehow her losses did not seem to overshadow her triumphs and vice versa. She acknowledged both stories. They seemed to exist alongside of each other, perhaps giving energy, meaning, and depth to her life. Without further delay, I sent off a note to her asking how exactly she had "triumphed" over waking up in a hospital with no hearing? It was essentially the same question she had asked me after my lecture.

Her reply came the next day:

I had to take a year's leave of absence from college to recuperate. I was living at home with my parents, going to physical rehab and a host of doctors. I remember when it first really hit on a deep, visceral level that I was deaf and that I was going to be deaf forever. It was the middle of the night, about a year after I left the hospital. A terrible nightmare about suffocating in a plastic bag had just woken me up. My heart was pounding and my whole body was covered with sweat. Without any hesitation, I immediately went straight to my parents' room, like I was a little girl again.

For a minute I stopped in my tracks and stood there noticing how soundly they were sleeping and how very peaceful they looked, but there was no question in my mind that they would want me to disturb all of that. So I shook them out of their sound, peaceful sleep and told them about my nightmare. We all knew what it meant.

My mother held me; I felt her body spasm and we both began to cry. She began to stroke my hair. My dad was sitting up in bed with one hand on my mom's shoulder and the other one on mine. He was crying, too. I felt real close to both of them that night. It was the first time that we really allowed ourselves to openly feel and express with each other the pain and tragedy of what had happened. None of us got any more sleep that night.

As the sun rose, my dad suggested we take a walk. I walked between my parents—hand in hand—just like I used to do as a kid, along the same paths in the woods that we had walked so many times before. The sun came up over the trees, through the mist, exposing the splendor of greens and other colors of the woods. Although I guess it may sound corny to you, it was an epiphany for me.

We were quiet for a long time. My dad was the first one to break the silence. As we sat down on a triangularly arranged group of rocks, he said very gently and lovingly, "You know, pumpkin (his pet-name for me), you'll get through this. You're going to have a full, happy and very successful life—but not without some blood, sweat, and tears. You never have to shut us out from any of that."

We all began to cry again and we sat there for a very long time. The mist was gone and the sun by this time radiated through the trees. I think that moment was the closest I've ever felt to my mom and dad. It was then I knew that everything would be okay.

While I read Carol's letter for the ump-teenth time, Sue in the chapter titled "Dear Mom and Dad," came to mind. The bond that Carol had with her parents was what Sue had resigned herself to only fantasizing about via imagined letter writing and psychodrama. Carol's parents had somehow been able to resist being consumed by their own grief so that they were able to help Carol with hers.

This theme was also explored in a biographical movie about C.S. Lewis's life entitled "Shadowlands." When his wife died, also leaving behind her young son, Lewis (Anthony Hopkins) became immobilized, that is, until his brother confronted him with "Your grief would be your business except now there's a child involved." He then pleaded with Lewis to "Talk to the boy." Later when C.S. Lewis shared his grief with the young boy, they cried together and their healing was made possible.

Carol's experience also made me think of author and poet Maya Angelou who, in her book *I Know Why the Cage Bird Sings,* described her childhood trauma of being sexually abused. For more than five years afterward, she did not talk at all. She described how her healing began in the company of "Mrs. Flowers":

> Childhood's logic never asks to be proved (all con-
> clusions are absolute). I didn't question why Mrs.
> Flowers had singled me out for attention. . . . All I
> cared about was that she had made tea cookies for
> me and read to me from her favorite book. It was
> enough to prove that she liked me.[2]

I began my next e-mail to Carol describing how touched
I was by her story. It was my hope to be able to give to my
own children that kind of gift in their times of crises. I also
expressed my wish to Carol that she share with me how she
had become so resilient. Can resilience be consciously created? Although I did not know what she wanted out of our
correspondence, I openly hoped that we could share our
two very different perspectives of acquired hearing loss and
perhaps create a more evolved and complete story of how,
when, and why things go well.

In that letter, I included some recent research on resilience theory for her comments. The conclusion of the research was that resilient children typically develop a close
early bond with at least one significant adult—sometimes a
family member, mentor, or other surrogate care-giver.[3]
Carol's story of walking into her parents room feeling assured that "they would want me to disturb their peace" exemplified this necessary ingredient beautifully.

"Psychologists should spend more time studying resilience instead of pathologizing or blaming victims of various misfortunes," Carol responded. She was already quite
familiar with "the literature pathologizing deaf people" and
had little use for professionals who, in her words, "want to
make a buck by diagnosing deaf people as mentally ill and
therefore in need of their treatment."

She then emphasized how vital it is to have "strong, nurturing, supportive connections with others." As an example, she wrote that she and her parents had begun taking

sign language classes about one year after her traumatic hearing loss, in her words, "once the dust had settled."

She elaborated:

> The class taught us some signs to use as an additional communication tool (although it was very cumbersome and awkward at first). More importantly, for that particular period of time in my life, our attending the class had become a special ritual whereby my parents showed me that they understood my needs. It felt very supportive and loving.

It was interesting to me that Carol emphasized the supportive, relational aspects of that class rather than what benefits it would have to ease the communication with her parents. Those benefits would come later as they became more comfortable with sign language.

That ritual not only forged a closer bond between Carol and her parents but also allowed for new relationships to be created with another important group of supportive people—Deaf adults. At first, this occurred in the context of their class, as the teacher had invited several "visiting Deaf professors." Then Carol and her parents attended several Deaf community events, at the recommendation of their teacher. There they made informal contacts, and soon they actively sought out Deaf adults, some of whom had been born deaf and some of whom had adventitious hearing losses, now inviting them to their home for dinner and conversation.

> We wanted to know how they succeeded in their lives. We wanted real life role models to prove that deafness didn't mean failure. My parents and I sometimes chuckle about the advice we got from professionals: 'It's too soon to meet Deaf people,' they warned; you need to go through the grieving process first.' We nodded our heads politely, but

kept on doing what we knew was right for us. It's important for professionals to have their theories, but they should listen to people more.

That hit a familiar nerve! I thought of Mary, in the chapter titled "Between Two Worlds," who kept trying to explain to me how I did not take her needs as a hard-of-hearing person seriously. It took the juxtaposition of our sessions with my realizing how my agency had ignored the needs of our hard-of-hearing conference audience to make what Mary had been trying to tell me "get through my head." Norma in the chapter titled "Presbycusis, Mortality, and Brussels Sprouts," also came to mind. She needed her family and therapist to understand the importance of her choosing how to live her life and experience her death.

I keep relearning the balancing act of being guided by both what an individual says about him/herself and what a theory says about a group of individuals. Theories offer only questions, also known as hypotheses. The individual must be the ultimate guide.

Carol then wrote about the abundance of support she received from her current family:

I'll never forget when I was introduced to Richard, several years after my accident. He seemed like a male version of Katherine Hepburn—tender and strong. We were married six months later. He and I have always worked very hard to be there for each other—to understand and be sensitive to each other's needs. On a weekly basis—for the most part—we go out and be together as a couple. It feeds our relationship.

Although Rick is hearing, he never minimizes what I have to go through every day, nor is he patronizing. When our children try to exclude me by putting their hands over their mouths or looking the other way—to play him off against me—he always insists that they face me and talk slowly so I can lip-read them. Rick and the kids have also taken a number of sign language classes by themselves and with me. Although they're far from fluent, they know several signs and finger-spell fairly well. So I don't always have to rely on lip-reading them. It's also nice that, when I have Deaf friends over, Rick and the kids can join in the conversation.

The Deaf and Hearing Worlds

I was curious about Carol's affiliations with the hearing world—including her family and work—and the Deaf world. In my next e-mail, I included an earlier version of the chapter now titled "Between Two Worlds" and asked her for any personal reactions.

Her response was rich in imagery:

> For me, I don't imagine myself caught in a tug-of-war between the two worlds like Mary in your paper. I imagine myself standing still, sometimes looking at the Deaf world, other times at the hearing world—while, all the time, holding hands with my family and a few intimate friends—both Deaf and hearing. I'm reasonably comfortable functioning in both worlds.

In my next e-mail, I asked her more specifically what "world(s)" of people with hearing losses were included in her image. They go by different names such as culturally Deaf, deaf, hearing-impaired, deafened, persons with acquired hearing losses, etc.

Carol's response came a few days later:

> Mike, now you're sounding like a Sociologist! (Smile). Of course, there are many so-called worlds.

Initially, I immersed myself in Deaf culture and the Deaf community. I took ASL classes, got additional tutoring, and socialized with many culturally Deaf people who remain my friends to this day. After a while, I found myself gravitating more to deafened adults. It seemed that we had more shared experiences, more in common.

Maybe I should revise my image (there's never enough time!) to show me walking in and out of the Deaf community but mostly "hanging out" in the world of people like me who have lost their hearing later in life. We're called Late-Deafened Adults.

I'm proud to say that I'm fluent in sign language— some ASL but mostly Pidgin Sign English. In addition, I continually learn about all the latest ALD's (Assistive Listening Devices), like FM systems, audio-loops, etc. My audiologist—who is very knowledgeable and supportive—keeps me up to date, often sending me journal articles. I wear digital hearing aids which, although they cost a fortune, are well worth it.

A few days later, I asked Carol "Do you have thoughts or feelings that you can reveal only to other deafened persons?" I suppose it was a loaded question since I am not deafened.

Her e-mail response contained miscellaneous content and ended with

Regarding your last question, now you're acting like a Psychologist again. Yes, there are certainly some things that I can discuss only with people like me who have lost their hearing. I'm really sorry, but you have to be deafened to understand. I hope you're okay with that. Gotta go now and grade some papers. Take care.

What did Carol mean? As much as I very much understood her sentiment—for I know well that there are certain
things only "like-others" can understand—I must admit
that—on an emotional level—I felt a bit indignant, maybe
even a bit hurt, but I did not want to show that part of me
to Carol. The advantage of pen-pal correspondence is that
you can pick your words carefully.

I responded simply with "Of course, I'm okay with that.
No problem. I respect your wishes if you don't want to tell
me about a private experience, but, assuming you're comfortable doing so, would you try to explain your identity as
a deafened person to me?"

Carol started her next e-mail with "I'm glad you don't
have hurt feelings. It's amazing how many people do!"

"It is amazing," I would affirm in my next note.

Carol continued:

That was one of the biggest fights Rick and I have
had. He felt like I was shutting him out of an intimate part of my life.

A critical part of my journey toward understanding
what it means to be a deafened person is to be with
other people who have also lost their hearing later
in life. Although I also need people different than
me, i.e., hearing and culturally Deaf people, African-
Americans, Asians, etc., I also very much need other
people like me. Attending A.L.D.A. conventions, for
example, feeds me in a way that nobody or nothing
else can. In a way, it feels like going home.

With that "extended peer family," I can begin a sen-
tence and have another complete it. Although Rick
and I often have that magic together (naturally it
comes in cycles as sometimes we're not in sync at
all), there's a special kind of 'mind reading' magic
that happens when I'm among my peers.

She ended with "But most of my professional life is in the hearing world."

"How do you do it?" I asked.

When I go to lectures in the community or at the university, I often get an interpreter, although I prefer real-time captioning. For my larger classes at the university, I always use a sign language interpreter, and my students have learned some basic communication rules—i.e., speaking clearly, making sure I'm able to look at them and talking one at a time. That makes life easier for me.

My deafness forced me to give up some control that I at least thought I had. In the old days, I would not be satisfied having attended a lecture, for example, if I did not understand each and every word: 100 percent of all the information. Now—even with the best of support services—it is very rare for me to understand everything. If the interpreter's any good or the captioning stenographer is well trained, I may get seventy-five or eighty percent of what's going on. Often I have come to accept that, naturally depending on the importance of the information.

It's a balancing act between accepting those imposed limitations which are, in fact, inevitable verses prematurely and unnecessarily giving up control and power.

My response a day later: "Thank you for your poignant description of your internal dialogue even when you have the best of accommodations. You make the external part of getting those support services sound so easy! Forgive my cynicism, but whomever pays for them doesn't just say 'Oh sure, no problem: Just tell me what accommodations you need.' Do they?"

"Of course not," came her reply. "It's a ongoing battle requiring a constant outflow of energy. I continue to be dumbfounded by how some people just don't get it or don't even want to get it."

Carol then elaborated that the most difficult part of being deaf is "not deafness per se, it's the damn insensitivity of much of the world. Most people put up a good front about having compassion and striving for equality until it inconveniences them in some way."

She then listed many instances of job discrimination that she has had to overcome. She went on to describe one example in her private life:

> Even Rick's family at Thanksgiving makes absolutely no effort to include me by speaking slowly, etc., even at the outset. (Whereas most people at social gatherings include you in conversations at the beginning until they get tired.) Even some of the younger kids sometimes poke fun at me when I can't lip-read them correctly. It hurts!

> Although that's a relatively benign and trivial example, similar kinds of insensitivity happen all the time in other more important 'arenas,' i.e., at community events, town meetings (I'm active in local politics), and at various university meetings. I always have to fight and fight real hard for accommodations. It's peoples' cruelty that 'traumatizes me' more than anything else.

Carol included a quotation from Gallaudet University Professor Allen Sussman, who is himself Deaf, that she had used when teaching a class on "The Sociology of Oppression"

> It is a rare deaf person who has not as a child been ostracized, ridiculed, and denigrated by non-disabled children. Such memories are painfully poignant.[4]

I returned a quotation by Cornel West from his book *Race Matters*. He is a Harvard University Professor and is himself African-American:

> I waited and waited and waited. After the ninth taxi refused me, my blood began to boil. The tenth taxi refused me and stopped for a kind, well-dressed, smiling female fellow citizen of European descent. As she stepped in the cab, she said, "This is really ridiculous, is it not?"
>
> Ugly racial memories of the past flashed through my mind. Years ago, while driving from New York to teach at Williams College, I was stopped on fake charges of trafficking cocaine. When I told the police officer I was a professor of religion, he replied, "Yeah, and I'm the Flying Nun. Let's go, nigger!"... Those memories cut like a merciless knife at my soul as I waited on that godforsaken corner.[5]

"What do you do with your rage?" I asked.

"Didn't you once tell me that 'one should seek to better understand it and then share those insights with supportive others?' (smile). That's what I do, but I don't stop there. Insight and validation aren't enough. It all has to lead to empowerment, to standing up for your rights!"

Carol then included a quotation from Psychiatrist Judith Herman's book *Trauma and Recovery* that I had recommended to her earlier:

> Helplessness and isolation are the core experiences of psychological trauma. Empowerment and re-connection are the core experiences of recovery.[6]

In her next e-mail, she then elaborated:

> Empowerment of women in this society is often frowned upon and viewed by men (and some

women) as "bitchiness." So we have to work doubly hard at it, both to show our strength to others and to feel good about it ourselves.

I have earned a reputation for refusing to let others dominate or oppress me. I'm not known for taking a lot of shit. For example, remember when I told you about being treated like a non-person by Rick's family at Thanksgiving? You know what I do now?

Rick and I came up with the strategy of my bringing a book to read when things like that would happen. First I plop myself down. Then I open up a good book, one I make sure is a thick hardcover. It makes everyone incredibly uncomfortable. Then, more often than not, people notice and include me in their conversations. If they don't, I catch up on my reading!

Carol's assertiveness and tenacity reminded me of a description of Jack Ashley, a British Parliament member who had suddenly become deaf, provided by his wife, Pauline Ashley:

Self confidence is key . . . What they [friends and colleagues] have noticed is that Jack does not feel inferior because of deafness, and therefore he never behaves in the slightly humbled way that the struggle to understand so often induces in the deaf person. With a temperament that is a mix of aggression, warmth, and humor, he is constitutionally incapable of allowing others to dominate him. (p. 81)[7]

Both Carol and Jack had enough self-esteem to "refuse to take shit."

Spirituality

Many weeks had passed since I last corresponded with Carol. One night I was rehashing in my mind a particularly moving session with Eric (see the chapter "Pockets of Gold") in which he had described his questioning of God. Many people ask a version of "why" after experiencing major losses or other calamities. I wondered about Carol, as we had never discussed this topic. I made time to e-mail her before putting my kids to bed.

Carol's response:

> After my accident, I spent a lot of time thinking about God and talking about spirituality with my parents and minister. Why did God allow this to happen? Did I deserve the accident—like they taught us in Sunday School? "Tell the righteous it shall be well with them, for they shall eat the fruit of their deeds. Woe to the wicked, it shall be ill with him, for what his hands have done shall be done to him." (Isaiah 3:10–11)

> Did God have some divine purpose or plan in mind that we mortals couldn't comprehend? Was the accident a test of my faith? (A new sequel: "Job meets Carol."). Was my suffering designed to somehow repair a flaw in my personality or character? Did God do this to me because She knew I could endure it? I had these questions and many more.

> Now I no longer hold God accountable. My understanding of God has changed dramatically from an anthropomorphic magician to a kind of "energy force." I still very much need a sense of the divine. God, for me, is the essence of connecting to the universe. I often experience "the divine" while among nature—or by the rhythmic movements of the waves, during special moments with my kids, by meditation, or often in church. That definition of God continues to help me immensely and is one cornerstone of my life, but I've come to learn that that God cannot

keep me out of trouble or prevent bad things from happening.

God, it seems, is "something" many of us need, although its definitions may change. It reminds me of Woody Allen's parable about relationships: "This guy goes to a psychiatrist and says, 'Doc, uh, my brother's crazy. He thinks he's a chicken.' And the doctor says, 'Well, why don't you turn him in?' And the guy says, 'I would, but I need the eggs.'"[8]

If There Were a Magic Pill. . . ?

It was probably only a matter of time until I asked Carol the "magic pill" question. Tonight, it seemed particularly relevant, as I found myself ruminating about a session I had that day with Robert (see the chapter "Changing the Rules of Trivial Pursuit"). He had told me that his "dark cloud" would instantly disappear if there were a magic pill that would make him hearing again.

I asked Carol for her reaction to the well-known interview with I. King Jordan [the first Deaf President of Gallaudet University] on the TV show "60 Minutes."*

> His answer very much affirms how I view my own identity. I wouldn't want to become hearing again, even if I could. It's not that I don't miss hearing many things (I do!)—like my daughter's singing recital and Rock and Roll, to mention only a couple—but my identity is now as a deaf person, specifically a late-deafened person. That's who I am now. My identity, like my spirituality, has become another cornerstone for me, one that continues to give meaning and purpose to my life and work.

---

*When Meredith Vieira asked "If there was a magic pill to make you hearing and you could swallow it, would you take it?" I. King Jordan responded with "Would you take a pill to become white? Would you take a pill to become a man?"

But I don't think deaf people who wish they were hearing are maladjusted. Some of my deaf friends and colleagues would rather be hearing; other deaf people like me cannot imagine it any other way. There are many modes of being in this world.

I guess whether you are "adjusted" or "maladjusted," in part, depends on how much you let the "I wish I was . . ." statements dominate your life. We all have, in the words of author Judith Viorst, necessary losses that we must reconcile as part of our maturational process. For Carol, the sorrow of her hearing loss was balanced by what purpose and meaning it had given her.

A Therapist's Odyssey

One evening, I arrived home to a short and to-the-point e-mail from Carol: "Enough about me. How has listening to peoples' stories of trauma and oppression affected you?"
I was tempted to respond with "I'm very sorry but you have to be a therapist to understand," but it would have been a wee bit infantile. Instead, I answered her short question with a long treatise, as the topic was one that I had been thinking a lot about.

> Carol, you asked a very relevant question which I hope this rather detailed note will answer. There are indeed hazards to empathy! Any helping professional knows too well that the effects of trauma and oppression are contagious. I have been particularly moved by Elie Wiesel's stories which illustrate four possible Vicarious Trauma reactions to observing oppression: that of an Oppressor, a Victim, a Bystander, and a Witness.[9]

> An *Oppressor.* Although it may be politically incorrect to acknowledge that we oppress another, it's something we all do, at least to some degree, when

we're in pain. A therapist's pain is a necessary arti-fact of "empathic atunement" with a client's experi-ence of powerlessness. A natural reaction is to attempt to make another's pain go away, but, in many cases, our bubble is burst and we become frus-trated, anxious, and often feel inadequate. To shield ourselves from these uncomfortable feelings, we may project them onto the client. We pathologize them—oppress them. I am guilty of this when I "hold on too tightly" to my diagnosis of a person, be-lieving it to represent the only truth as opposed to simply one of many ways to understand that person, and a crude one at that.

A *Victim*: Or we may proudly offer ourselves to our clients as sacrificial lambs, as compensation for when other hearing people have oppressed them. Addi-tionally, since many helping professionals have been parentified, i.e., their parents expected them to act like adults at too young an age—or have been abused as children, we may identify with the oppressed. Rather than take care of our own emotional needs, we may unwittingly come to rely on helping others to gain self respect. Sooner or later, we succumb to its insidious, debilitating effects. I am thankful to my wife for reminding me when I—more regularly than I would like to admit—fall into this trap.

A *Bystander*: Those who routinely witness oppression may unwittingly erect a shell of protective numb-ness. The result is so-called "compassion fatigue": "I have a job to do and that's all that matters."10 One example was when I found myself daydreaming about lunch instead of focussing on the overwhelm-ing sadness of a client's story (see the chapter "Es-caping the Dungeon of Oppression").

A *Witness*: Bearing witness to the oppression of another is to grapple—both privately and publicly—
with how and why that oppression exists; to question
whether one is complicit in perpetuating it, and to
do one's part to minimize it. As a witness, we are not
only vicariously traumatized but also more profoundly transformed. In my case, like many others, I
was forced to give up a naive, but developmentally
necessary, innocence about the invariable goodness
of humanity.

"Does that answer your question?" I asked in closing.

Only a few hours after I had sent her that message,
Carol sent me the following one-sentence response: "Stop
over intellectualizing and give me a more personal answer
to my question, please. (Smile.)"

I responded in jest that no one had given me that feedback before. Over intellectualizing is a professional liability.
Second try, two days later: a more personal response.

For me, being a psychotherapist has meant the best
of times and the worst of times. Often I feel proud
and confident that I'm helping people remove whatever obstacles lie in their path to a better life. It en-
riches me too, as our collaboration and dialogue
evolves to encompass a wider range of what it means
to be human. I feel very lucky and privileged to learn
first-hand what lies behind a person's persona, what
that person would not dare show in public, perhaps
not even to him/herself.

While the outcome of a person's therapeutic odyssey
seldom surprises me (as I've witnessed it many times),
I very much continue to be profoundly amazed by its
unique twists and turns. I am thankful for that.

At these times, I cannot imagine doing anything different to give meaning and purpose to my life. Those are the best of times.

At other times, my clarity evaporates—or perhaps it was all a delusion? I become overwhelmed, even a bit angry, with the complexity of human beings. Some people either can't or won't get better for a variety of charted and uncharted reasons. Sometimes the best map won't guide you.

As a psychotherapist, I can only collect stories from clients, make some theoretical sense out of them, and attempt to be helpful. On my good days, it feels like a worthy endeavor; on my bad days, it feels lacking.

I often long for the certainty that I imagine my auto mechanic has. It would all be so clear: clean the carburetor, grind the valves, adjust the timing belt. It would be irrelevant whether or not a piston engine is motivated or ready to change, and there would be no "family-member cars" to consider while doing repairs.

People, however, aren't cars. All too often, The Grand, Therapeutic Odyssey seems like it's going nowhere fast, or I find myself reacting to a person in front of me as if he or she embodied a host of significant others in my life—perhaps my mother, father, a mentor, one whom I had feared, adored, or respected. (Auto mechanics also don't have to worry about countertransference.)

Then there is the omnipresent danger of my becoming too "other-focused" rather than "self-focused." My caring about and needing to help another person can easily become a necessity, an obsession. *Codependence.*

I have also found that doing therapy can become quite lonely, as it's largely one-way. Connected to every utterance out of my mouth (or hands) there is a part of my cerebral cortex which, by necessity, must always ask "Are you being helpful right now?" Receiving consultation, my own psychotherapy or peer group support, becomes a necessity for both my own survival and continued effectiveness to those who seek my help.

Writing has also become a necessary labor of love. I write out of my own need to put into words some of the most important things I have come to believe as well as what I'm in the process of trying to figure out. Equally as important—or perhaps more so—I have long realized my need for another to react to me, whether positively or negatively—whatever! In some ways it doesn't matter. For that dialog is an essential part of my defining who I am.

That's why I have come to cherish our long-term conversation so much. I don't have to try to help you, just as you don't have to try to help me, but we help each other nonetheless. I thank you for that.

I ended by offering to send Carol a treatise on counter-transference theory. She responded that same day with "very funny."

————

Carol and I continue our correspondence, sometimes quite frequently, other times after weeks or months pass. We exchange our personal stories and invite the other to embellish them—to question, critique, and challenge. Through our intimate dialogue, our stories have evolved to a richness, depth, and complexity that is "more" than each of our stories taken individually. "The Gestalt is more than the sum of its parts."

I have learned some important lessons about strength, courage, and resiliency from Carol—much like what I have learned from those for whom I provided therapy. An important point: It is not that the psychotherapy clients in this book are dysfunctional, while Carol is functional. The gold and dragons contained within all of our shadows are similar in form, although different in content. Per the title of an album by the comedy group Firesign Theatre, "We're All Bozos on This Bus."

Another story may further illustrate this point. A group of experienced psychotherapists were viewing videotapes of a functional family and a dysfunctional family. In response to the functional family, the therapists volunteered an impressive array of the obvious as well as the subtle indications of adjustment and psychological health. Similarly, in response to the dysfunctional family, the therapists perceptively listed numerous indications of maladjustment and psychopathology. Then an embarrassing thing happened. They realized that they had mislabeled the videotapes! The tape that was labeled "Functional Family" was actually the dysfunctional family and vice versa.

So how, when, and why did things go well for Carol? She was not born resilient. Rather, she was lucky enough to have had some key supports at critical times in her life. Subsequently, they became incorporated into her psyche as "internal guides" which continually helped her more comfortably accept support from others as well as have the courage to meet head-on various life challenges, including cultural insensitivity.

Over the past year, I had mentioned to Carol that I was writing this book. It was largely her idea for me to include a chapter with some of the relevant content from our correspondence. In her words, "it would elucidate to both consumers and professionals that acquired hearing loss does not mean succumbing to an unfulfilled life."

One night I e-mailed Carol and asked her what she would like to title our chapter. I suggested "An Inspirational

Voice from Cyberspace." Whereas she typically responded to questions within days, this time it took her a couple of weeks. The thoughtfulness of her reply explained the delay:

> My thoughts about the title for "our" chapter reflect the thoughts I have for a title of my life. It has contained plenty of wonderful, happy, and sometimes even blissful times, and it has contained a lot of pain and loss. However, despite all the adversity that I have faced, I feel very lucky—even blessed—to have inner strength and self-love. These I have earned from hard work and from the love and support of my family. Although my life has not been smooth (nobody's life is), my path has been a lot smoother than it could have been. Hopefully the title could convey that message.

Carol has come to be one of the more important people in my life since our correspondence began five years ago. However, I would not recognize her even if I bumped into her. Her e-mail address, however, I know by heart.

Notes

1. Hemingway, E. (1929). *A farewell to arms* (p. 239). New York: Charles Scribner's Sons.

2. Angelou, M. (1969). *I know why the caged bird sings* (p. 85). New York: Bantam Books.

3. Butler, K. (1997). The anatomy of resilience. *Family Therapy Networker*, 22–31.

4. Sussman, A. E. (1976). Attitudes toward deafness: Psychology's role—past, present, and potential. In F. B. Crammette & A. B. Crammette (Eds.), *VII World Congress of the World Federation of the Deaf* (p. 10). Washington, DC: National Association of the Deaf.

5. West, Cornel. (1993). *Race matters*. Boston, MA: Beacon Hill Press.

6. Herman, J. L. (1992). *Trauma and recovery* (p. 197). New York: Basic Books.

7. Ashley, P. K. (1985). Deafness in the family. In H. Orlans (Ed.), *Adjustment to adult hearing loss*. San Diego, CA: College-Hill Press.

8. McCann, G. (1990). *Woody Allen* (p. 113). New York: Polity Press.

9. Brown, R. M. (1989). *Elie Wiesel: Messenger to all humanity—revised edition*. Notre Dame, IN: Notre Dame Press.

10. Figley, C. R. (1995). *Compassion fatigue: Coping with secondary traumatic stress disorder in those who treat the traumatized*. New York: Brunner/Mazel.